Kettlebells for 50+

Kettlebells for 50+

Safe and Customized Programs
for Building & Toning Every Muscle

Dr. Karl Knopf

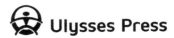
Ulysses Press

Published in the United States by
Ulysses Press
P.O. Box 3440
Berkeley, CA 94703
www.ulyssespress.com

ISBN: 978-1-61243-046-1
Library of Congress Control Number 2012931428

Printed in Canada by Webcom

10 9 8 7 6 5 4 3 2 1

Acquisitions: Kelly Reed
Managing editor: Claire Chun
Editor: Lily Chou
Proofreader: Elyce Berrigan-Dunlop
Indexer: Sayre Van Young
Production: Judith Metzener
Front cover design: what!design @ whatweb.com
Photographs: © Rapt Productions
Models: Fred Brevold, Rob Harrison, Karl Knopf, Toni Silver

Distributed by Publishers Group West

Please Note
This book has been written and published strictly for informational purposes, and in no way should be used as a substitute for actual instruction with qualified professionals. The author and publisher are providing you with information in this work so that you can have the knowledge and can choose, at your own risk, to act on that knowledge. The author and publisher also urge all readers to be aware of their health status and to consult health care professionals before beginning any health program.

contents

getting
started

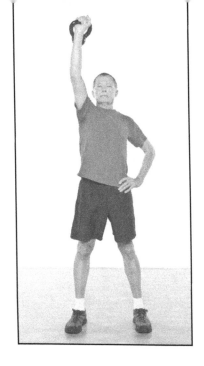

introduction

The fountain of youth has been discovered! However, it's not in a bottle, an injection or even a pill. It's found in a daily dose of sensible physical activity. While many 50+ people understand the importance of aerobic exercise, many neglect a critical component to successful aging—maintaining strength and power. Specifically, a lack of strength and power in our legs and trunk reduces our ability to attend to basic activities of daily living.

This weakness increases the risk of falling and reduces our independence. Using kettlebells is a great option to build strength and prevent sarcopenia, or age-related atrophy. A basic kettlebell exercise program will engage your legs, trunk and upper body and help you stay fit for life.

Kettlebells for 50+ invites everyone to incorporate kettlebell training into their lives. Although this book is similar to other kettlebell exercise books, it's also very different. As an adaptive physical education teacher for more than 35 years, I believe that the person and the purpose of the movement are more important than some prescribed movement pattern. For this reason, many of the exercises selected for this book have been adapted to better suit baby boomers, offering the most benefit and the least amount of insult to the vintage body. Any traditional kettlebell exercise that I felt compromised body mechanics or failed to have a functional purpose was not included. As I always say, "Train smart, not hard."

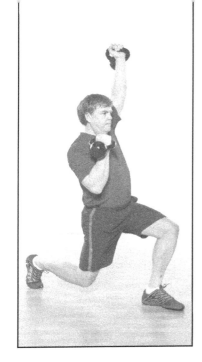

what is old is new again

The kettlebell, or *girya* in Russian, is a cast-iron weight that looks like a cannonball with a teapot handle (personally, I think the name should be "kettle*ball*" because of its shape). It's believed to have originated in the eastern European countries in the late 1800s, originally used as a past-time activity and as circus stunts by big burly men displaying feats of strength. As time progressed, people started to use the kettlebell as a method to improve strength and fitness. In the former Soviet Union, Olympic weightlifting coaches used kettlebells as a training device.

The kettlebell arrived in the United States in the early 1900s and was used by immigrants and, along with the medicine ball, was slowly introduced into boxing clubs as a training device. The kettlebell lost favor in the '70s when the fitness industry moved toward selectorized weight machines. It was at this time that Nautilus equipment became the rage and old-time medicine balls, club bells, dumbbells, barbells and kettlebells were replaced with shiny, cambered, belt-driven resistance-training equipment.

Forty years later, "old-school" training devices have come back into vogue. Today we see boot-camp training programs and shadow boxing put to music. Many personal trainers new to fitness think that push-ups, jumping jacks, squat thrusts and kettlebells are something very in-novative but most of us 50+ folks can say, "Been there, done that." For some of us, reintroducing kettlebells into our lives may be like visiting an old friend.

Kettlebells are part of the plyometric family, which includes exercises such as jumping, bounding, and throwing and catching weighted objects such as medicine balls or kettlebells. These movements involve rapid eccentric (lengthening) and concentric (shortening) actions.

Plyometric exercises have their roots in the 1960s, when they were first used in the Eastern Bloc countries to train their weightlifters and track-and-field athletes. A plyometric workout was, and still is, designed to improve explosive muscular power.

The reason the kettlebell is gaining favor again is that the motions involved in a kettlebell workout mimic activities of daily living much more than the unidirectional exercise machines seen in most gyms today. The kettlebell is used to perform dynamic exercises that foster power, agility, strength, flexibility and even aerobic fitness. The shape of the kettlebell places the center of gravity beyond the handle, which allows the bell to be thrown about easily, facilitating swing movements. Some versions of kettlebells include bags filled with steel shot, sand or adjustable weight plates. When used properly, kettlebells are a challenging and enjoyable adjunct to a standard total-body fitness program.

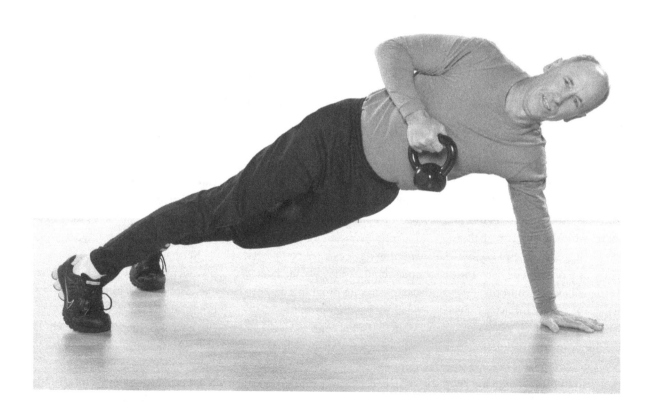

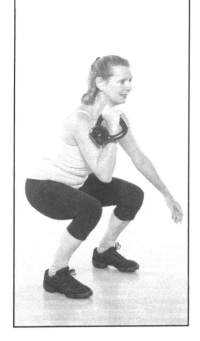

why use kettlebells?

Anyone who has exercised for any period of time has probably gotten stale, bored or burnt out with the same old routine. Kettlebells aren't a be-all and end-all piece of equipment, but they do offer a fabulous diversion and can be used alone in an exercise routine or integrated into an existing strength-training program. They can provide you with a comprehensive total-body workout that addresses strength, power, core stabilization, agility and hand-to-hand coordination as well as hand-eye coordination.

Kettlebells are basically odd-shaped weights with handles. The handle placement in relation to the weighted ball off-balances the load, creating an additional dynamic force when used. With this design, you can move in several planes and develop strength and power in the legs, lower back, grip and shoulders. We need to think of our body as a total kinetic chain unit, which means that what happens at one point affects something else down the chain. Just gripping the

bell handle engages the forearm muscles; swinging the bell from the floor to overhead engages the calf muscles, the butt muscles (gluteals), the back muscles and the shoulder muscles (deltoids), as well as many deep-lying muscles. To engage all those same muscles on an exercise machine would require at least three different machines.

Most traditional exercise programs performed with free weights or machines generally focus on one set of muscles at a

time. Kettlebell movements often target not only primary muscles but also the supporting muscle groups. Moves that involve momentum (such as swings) incorporate both acceleration and deceleration, but kettlebells can be used in a slow, controlled manner much like free weights. In this regard, when used correctly, the kettlebell is an ideal training device for all levels.

Most beginners need to start at the slow, controlled level and then progress to the more dynamic and advanced moves.

What are the advantages of kettlebells? They:

- are reasonably priced and last forever.
- are small and easy to store.
- are very adaptable—you can move them slowly, quickly and in almost any conceivable direction.
- are an efficient way to get a total-body workout in a shorter period of time.
- often better replicate functional activities of life and sport than exercise machines because of the incorporation of acceleration and deceleration.
- are a creative way to improve power and challenge the body.
- improve neuromuscular proprioception.
- improve body awareness and coordination.
- foster improved joint stabilization.
- are a fun and challenging diversion from the same old push-and-pull weight machines.

But the real beauty of a kettlebell workout is that it can replicate activities of daily living. The key to aging successfully is to be able to perform the tasks necessary to live a functionally independent life. The kettlebell helps you to attain that goal by personalizing your routine for your particular needs. However, a kettlebell program requires practice and patience to learn the correct body mechanics. As with any exercise tool, kettlebells can cause injury if you proceed too quickly or perform moves incorrectly. Too often baby boomers have the mind-set that more is better, but proper execution and engaging the mind and the body are the key to a successful kettlebell workout.

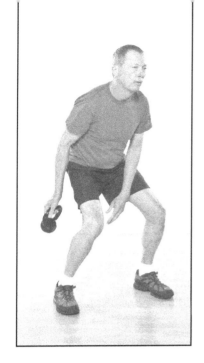

kettlebells for 50+ folks

The exercises in *Kettlebells for 50+* are practical and functional, and they're been tested and selected for the 50+ person based on years of experience. Some have been adapted from their original form to better serve the baby boomer's body. These movements will provide a complete and comprehensive workout of both the major and minor muscles of the body in a short amount of time. While more kettlebell exercises exist (as you may see in other books or on DVDs), many have been eliminated from this book to offer you the safest kettlebell approach possible.

The 50+ population runs the gamut from very frail to extremely fit. Some exercises in this book may be too difficult for some and too easy for others, but again this book is written for the middle group. Please seriously consider the movements and the size of the kettlebell you select with regard to your health status before you jump fully into a kettlebell workout. If you're an exercise novice, you should do well following the progression outlined in the programs section (page 25).

Most exercises performed with weight machines or free weights are done in a slow, controlled manner, whereas many kettlebell exercises can be done with momentum and in a freestyle manner. Note, however, that many of the exercises in this book utilize slower, controlled movements that are similar to using a dumbbell because they're considered more appropriate for the 50+ age group or someone starting a kettlebell program.

As you begin your workout, you'll find the exercises are more challenging than a basic dumbbell or conventional gym machine workout. Faster movements such as swings and catch-and-release exercises are more appropriate for stronger, well-conditioned exercisers who have a substantial foundation of strength training.

To train well, your mission is to train smart, not hard, and to not harm yourself. Please do not perform any movement beyond your skill set or fitness level. Too often baby boomers are in a hurry to get fit, but before they ever get fit they get hurt and quit. That might be okay for a 30-something who can recover quickly, but this could be devastating for a 50-something. Just getting up in the morning can be hazardous to your health, and any exercise program can be harmful as well if not performed correctly. So use caution when selecting any exercise method to gain fitness, especially if you have back or shoulder concerns.

If exercise is new to you, keep in mind that it'll take 12–16 weeks before you notice any change. It takes at least 3 months to establish a new habit. Don't quit before you have a chance to see results. If you think getting motivated is hard, staying motivated is just as hard. Make your fitness routine enjoyable and exciting by periodically changing your existing routine with different kettlebell exercises to enhance your desire to exercise. Find movements that match your personality as well as your physical strength and flexibility limits. Research on strength training shows that there's no absolute way to train to improve strength and muscle development. Always listen to your body and heed what it says—no one knows your body better than you.

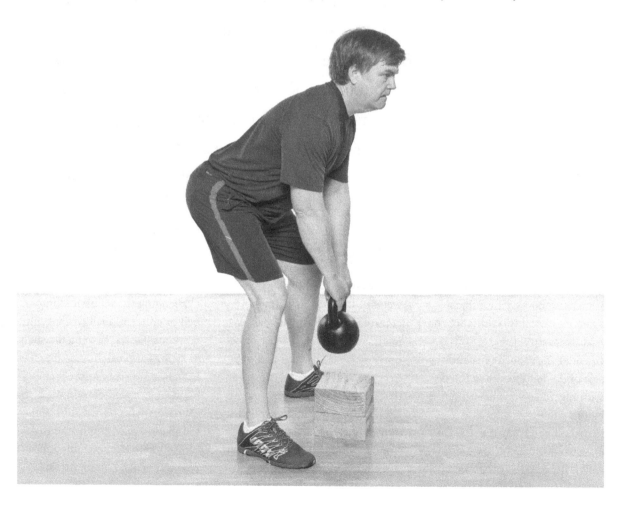

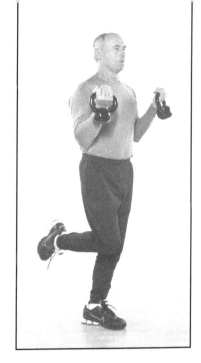

before you begin

While this book is designed for everyone, having a solid baseline of fitness, a basic understanding of resistive training concepts, and good coordination and body mechanics would be ideal in gaining the most from this book. As with any exercise program, it's prudent to consult your health care professional to see if you're healthy enough to perform this exciting and challenging workout. Take this book along with you to your doctor and ask him/her if your joints and cardiorespiratory system are able to accommodate this type of routine.

Safety

A kettlebell workout requires time to learn the movements correctly. Rushing into the program before you're ready is a recipe for aches and pain. In addition, you should never become complacent about a kettlebell workout: A kettlebell workout is a mind-body experience that requires your complete attention.

Some vintage athletes suffer from the "forever 21" complex, in which is they believe they can

still train like they did when they were 21. My training buddies and I call it "the older I get, the better I was" concept. They continue to work out intensely because they think their ability to exercise has not diminished too much with age, but their potential to get hurt while exercising has increased. Being over 50 is no reason to stop working out, but you need to exercise smart, not hard.

Kettlebell workouts are not an entry-level exercise routine, but

if you have a baseline of average or above average strength and muscular endurance, a kettlebell workout is an excellent addition to your training options. If you're new to exercise, start with the Introduction to Kettlebells workout on page 32; you may also want to review my *Weights for 50+* book before you begin a kettlebell program.

Too often 50+ folks are in a rush to get fit and often overestimate their ability or don't heed what their body is telling them. The result? Injury. Some of my clients tell me that they were an athlete before or did the exercise before so they can do it now, but they're wrong. Every 72 hours your body goes without exercise, it begins to de-condition. How many hours have elapsed since you last lifted weights? Note also that there's a concept of specificity of training, which means being fit for one activity doesn't necessarily carry over to another activity. So if you're a runner or tennis player, you may not be in kettlebell shape.

Learn the difference between good pain and bad pain. If you have a new pain or a pain that isn't going away, seek medical attention. Pain in the joint is generally bad pain, while muscle soreness generally isn't so bad. We all have our own threshold for pain. Don't ever mask the pain with drugs. The best recommendation is to train, don't strain and make movement fun!

Lastly, what you wear and where you do your kettlebell workout is important. You don't want to wear clothes that your hand(s) can get caught on while swinging the kettlebell and throw you off balance. It may sound silly to say, but once you've decided on your workout spot, spread your arms and legs and check out the area around you.

Is there ample space for you to throw a kettlebell around? Let people know that you're going to be doing your kettlebell workout so that no one walks in behind you and gets hit in the face. I don't want to hear that a flying kettlebell was a cause of an injury. Train safe!

Preventing Injuries

We've all heard the old saying that an ounce of prevention is worth a pound of cure, and that's important to keep in mind when it comes to our health. We all know that maintaining our cars will prevent a major breakdown. We should care for our bodies the same way.

Improper training and overtraining are common problems for some 50+ folks. Rather than implement the outdated exercise slogan "No pain, no gain," we should focus on "Motion is the lotion to the joints and the tonic to the brain." Overtraining is a major problem for highly active 50+ fitness participants. Overtraining occurs as a result of dramatically increasing training periods with high-volume or high-intensity workouts. There are both psychological manifestations of overtraining as well as physiological manifestations of overtraining: increased pain, reduced desire to train, loss of appetite, difficulty concentrating. Ask your doctor if your blood

KETTLEBELL CAUTIONS

Plyometric exercises are safe if used with common sense. The National Strength and Conditioning Association suggests the following safety guidelines:

- Plyometric exercises require more recovery time, so make sure to rest at least one day between workouts.
- Don't do kettlebell exercises when distracted or fatigued.
- Wear proper footwear and choose proper flooring.
- Warm up properly.
- Follow proper progressions: Learn less-intense and less-complex moves before trying more complex ones.

pressure and joints can handle a series of kettlebell exercises.

You don't necessarily need to work hard to gain results; mild to moderate intensity is ideal for health and function. The problem is finding the correct dose to get the ideal response. What's moderate for one person may be too vigorous for another, what's easy for someone may be hard for someone else. Re-assess your kettlebell routine if you have any increased joint discomfort or muscle soreness. Any pain that exceeds mild soreness means you're overdoing it and risking injury. It doesn't mean quit—just back off. Follow the 2-hour rule: If you have an increase in any pain 2 hours post-exercise, you've done too much.

A kettlebell workout, which may involve quick, ballistic moves, is unlike most other weight-training programs that many of us have done. While you may be very fit and well-trained, these exercises require time on task to learn proper form and pace. If you hasten the learning curve, you'll only invite problems later. Learn your joints' pain-free range of motion before engaging in kettlebell training. Once you earn the right to perform swings and other dynamic movements, focus on learning how to decelerate the kettlebell's motion before momentum takes you past your safe range of motion.

Here are a dozen simple guidelines to prevent a fitness injury.

Perform a thermal warm-up before starting. A warm-up increases the blood flow to the muscles, which in turn increases body temperature and facilitates flexibility. Generally, a good warm-up includes doing gentle, rhythmic moves such as walking and light cycling for 5–10 minutes prior to your exercise session.

Stretch properly after your kettlebell workout to maintain flexibility and prevent post-workout soreness. The best time to stretch is after a workout, when the muscles are warm. Move the joints only in patterns they're designed to move in. (More details can be found in my *Stretching for 50+* book.)

Get in shape to play. Too many baby boomers think that just coming out to play will get them in shape to compete. Nothing is further from the truth. Design your workout to match the demands of your sport/activity. A total-body program that includes proper strength training, stretching and aerobic exercise are the basics.

Engage proper body mechanics. Using your body improperly can lead to an injury.

Avoid overtraining. If you're feeling more pain, reduced desire to train, loss of appetite, difficulty concentrating, or emotional instability, you may be suffering from overtraining. Back off—you may have reached a plateau. Changing your routine may help.

Obtain your ideal weight. For every pound of weight you lose, there's a 4-pound reduction in load placed upon the knee joint with each step. If you do the math, a 1-pound loss in weight would be 4,800 pounds less load placed on the knee for every mile walked. Less weight = less pressure = less load on the knee.

Choose the kettlebell exercise that's right for you. If you like challenging activities and fast-moving sports, select those kettlebell movements that test your coordination. If you like activities that require attention to detail, select slow, purposeful kettlebell movements.

Cross-train. Mixing up activities/sports on alternate days is a great way to avoid burnout and overtraining. Switch the kettlebell exercises around every week so that you're always doing something new and exciting. If you're training in another activity, you could, say, do a kettlebell workout every Wednesday to keep your workout alive.

Listen to your body. If something hurts and doesn't feel right, back off and rest.

Take care of yourself—seek prompt medical care for injuries. The sooner you see the doctor, the quicker you'll return to the fitness arena.

SIGNS TO PUT OFF EXERCISE

- You have muscle aches from a viral infection.
- Your systolic blood pressure is greater than 150 at rest and your diastolic exceeds 100 at rest, or your heart rate is greater than 100 at rest. Remember, a kettlebell workout is strenuous!
- Your joint is red, swollen, warm or painful.
- You're experiencing a new pain.
- You're having chest pains, heart flutters or any signs of a stroke or heart attack.
- You have swollen limbs.
- You have trouble breathing.

Take your time getting back into shape. Don't rush–haste makes pain!

Avoid being sedentary. If you rest, you rust.

Common Problem Areas

The areas most frequently injured in 50+ folks are the neck, low back, shoulder, knee, hips, elbow and ankle. Special attention should be paid when performing kettlebell exercises that involve these areas. Older athletes are far more likely to injure themselves while participating in a fitness program than younger people performing the same activity. The good news is that approximately 85% of sports injuries seen in the 50+ group are caused by overuse, which fortunately responds well to conservative treatment. The key is to train, don't strain!

Neck

Neck problems can occur when you swing the kettlebell without paying attention to proper neck posture. Any activity that causes excessive hyperextension (e.g., throwing your head back as you throw the bell overhead or doing any fast motions that take your neck out of a neutral position) should be eliminated. Always remember that what happens at one part of the kinetic chain affects another part of the kinetic chain. Thus, poor posture in the low back affects the neck region and vice versa.

Low Back

The majority of adults will experience back pain at some time in their life. It's critical to protect your back and keep it stabilized when performing kettlebell exercises. Learning neutral spine technique is extremely important and will help you avoid an injury. Any kettlebell exercise that involves forward flexion and rotation at the same time is a high-risk exercise, as is any move that creates excessive hyperextension of the low back. Use caution when doing any movements that bend or twist your spine sideways. Consider performing any questionable movements without a kettlebell first to see how your body responds. If you have a back problem, ask your health professional about specific exercises you should avoid.

Shoulder

Shoulder impingement is becoming an increasing concern for 50+ exercisers. Shoulder problems can develop with long periods of overhead or repetitive motions. Use caution when bringing your arms above your head. Stay alert and aware of how far back your arms go when doing movements—if your hands go past your line of sight, you may have taken your arms back too far. Swinging kettlebells too high with arms fully extended can aggravate shoulder problems and may possibly cause elbow problems as well. Avoid shrugging your shoulders up near your ears. Always warm up the shoulder joint prior to shoulder moves.

Knee

It's a good idea to keep "knees soft" when doing a kettlebell workout. Movements that hyperextend or twist the lower leg should be eliminated. Also, use caution when twisting your body with your feet planted—always move your hips, torso and shoulders as a unit. Try your best to keep your knees over your toes when squatting or lunging; your knees and toes should always point in the same direction when doing lunges. Another precaution is to avoid overflexion of the knee joint—this is why full squats and full quadriceps stretches (i.e., bringing the heel toward the butt) are not included in this book. If you're bow-legged, you have an increased risk of knee problems. Some recent research suggests that women jump and land differently than men, which places them at greater risk of knee injuries. Often females have an increased "Q" angle, which is the angle from the hip to the knee.

Hips

Known as the powerhouse joint of the body, the hip can have problems, from bursitis to a complicated hip fracture to referred pain from a pinched nerve. Hip problems can be brought on by overuse and improper body mechanics, from crossing your legs to jogging on one side of the road all the time. To prevent a hip problem, avoid performing deep squats in which your butt is lower than your knees, explosive plyometric moves or high-impact activities, deep lunges, and dynamic leg-spreading moves such as jumping jacks. If you experience any hip issues, consider seeing a health professional and try changing the intensity and frequency of your routine. You may also want to change the type of exercises you do and expand your rest cycle.

Elbows

The elbow joint is made up of three bones as well as bursas, ligaments and tendons. Tendinitis is a very common disorder often brought on by overuse. When doing strength training, pay attention to the angle that feels best for your elbow—often, a slight twist of the wrist will take stress off the elbow joint. Keeping your arm straight but not locked when doing kettlebell swings will lessen the load on the elbow joint as well. Avoid extreme movements, such as hyperextension and hyperflexion of the elbow joint. If you experience any elbow issues, consider seeing a health professional and try changing the intensity and frequency of your routine. You may also want to change the type of exercises you do and expand your rest cycle. Try using an ice pack on the elbow joint after your workout

Ankles and Feet

Pay attention to the way you stand when doing kettlebell exercises—avoid rolling your ankles too far left or right. Try to distribute the load over your whole foot. Stay mindful that the shoes you wear may affect your balance and ankle stability.

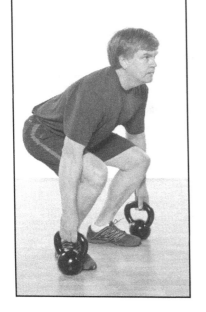

getting started

Performing kettlebell exercises is like hitting a tennis ball with a racquet. There's a big difference between hitting the ball in the sweet spot and just hitting the ball anywhere. If you perform the kettlebell move correctly, it just "feels" right. *Kettlebells for 50+* is about fluidity and grace, not grunt power. To achieve this, you'll need to find the right kettlebell (or two) for your workout.

Kettlebells by design are very different from dumbbells. You may notice that a 5-pound kettlebell feels very different than a 5-pound dumbbell. The influence of momentum is a major factor. It's critical to be comfortable with your particular range of motion. I often ask students to test out just the movement of the kettlebell exercise they'll be performing before even touching a kettlebell. Once they learn their safe range of motion, I have them use a light kettlebell to see how the element of momentum makes the movement feel different. Learning to accelerate and decelerate the kettlebell before

you select a training kettlebell load is critical.

Selecting Your Kettlebell

In the olden days, kettlebells were only available in black and weights ranged from heavy to very heavy. Today, kettlebells come in a variety of weights, styles and colors. Some kettlebells have rounded handles, others have more rectangular ones. Some are polished and smooth, others are rough. Traditionalists may prefer the black cast-iron version while others may prefer colorful, rubber-coated bells. Some trainers suggest that the unpainted handle version provides better control, but the selection of a

kettlebell is a personal issue. Find one that fits your hands and your training objectives.

Old-time kettlebell users refer to the weight in terms of *pood*, which is roughly 16 kilograms or 35 pounds. Nowadays, you'll find kettlebells weighing as little as 2 pounds to 165 pounds (75 kilograms). The weight you select depends on numerous variables, from the type of exercise you plan to perform, to your level of strength, to any underlying joint issues.

In general, I strongly suggest you start with a light kettlebell and increase the resistance slowly after seeing how your joints re-

Use this flow chart to help you determine the correct load for your exercise.

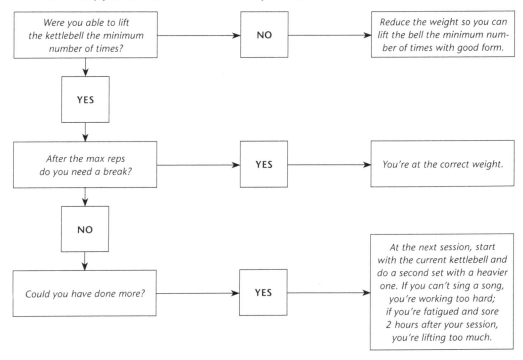

spond. Going heavier encourages you to compromise form and thus "cheat" to overcompensate for lack of strength and technique. In addition, the heavier you go, the more you increase your risk of injury. Don't let anyone say you should go heavier—listen to your inner trainer. If you plan to train regularly with kettlebells, you may need several different kettlebells to accommodate different types of moves (e.g., heavier for deadlifts, lighter for kneeling get-ups).

Some of my clients, before they purchase any kettlebells, try some of the basic kettlebell moves with standard dumbbells they already have. Many kettlebell exercises can be easily performed with a standard dumbbell. As you progress into the swing exercises, you'll know what size kettlebells to purchase. The cost of kettlebells has dropped significantly, with some sporting goods stores and department stores now selling sets in various ranges of weights.

Stances & Grips

Before you start your kettlebell workout, you should familiarize yourself with a few standard foot and handgrip positions. The way you grasp the kettlebell influences the types of motions you can perform. You should practice getting the feel of it before you commence a full-blown workout.

I'm a fanatic about proper body mechanics and posture, but your common sense will be a good determinant of what grip feels best for you for each exercise. Some authors tell you that there's only one way to grip the kettlebell for a specific exercise, but it's okay to adapt the position for your body. Remember, this is

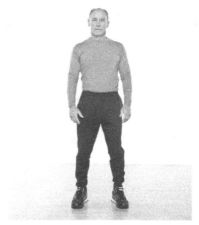

Regular stance

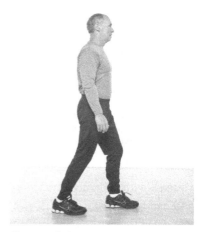

Staggered stance

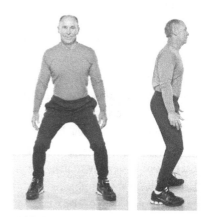

Athletic stance

an *adapted* kettlebell exercise book, so as long as you're enjoying the motion and it's not causing discomfort, go for it! This is your kettlebell program. However, it's extremely important that you have a solid grip of the kettlebell because once it gets moving, it's hard to hold on to!

It might be wise to invest in gloves or lifting chalk to improve your grip (gloves may prevent calluses, too). Switching grips mid-air is an option and requires good grip strength and hand-eye coordination, but it's not recommended until you're advanced. Note that hand switching is not necessary to improve strength and power.

Foot Positions

Wear shoes that provide you feedback with the ground and protect your foot should the kettlebell drop. Running shoes are not ideal for kettlebell training. A walking shoe, or some other flat footwear that provides lateral support and won't slip, would be a better choice.

Regular Stance: Stand erect with your feet shoulder-width apart and weight evenly distributed over both feet, shoulders relaxed, chest open and shoulder blades retracted (pulled back and down).

Staggered Stance: Step one foot forward and the other foot back, with your feet slightly

wider than hip-distance apart in a well-balanced lunge position. The knees should be slightly bent to provide stability and mobility. Engage your core. When performing exercises in this position, it's recommended that you perform one set with one leg forward and then switch sides in order to help maintain symmetry.

Athletic Stance (Shortstop): Stand with your feet a little wider than your shoulders and keep your back slightly rounded and ready for action.

Handgrips

Overhand (Palm Down): Place one hand on top of the handle as if you were grabbing a dumbbell to perform an exercise. This

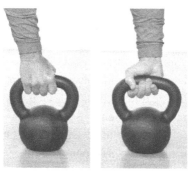

Left: Overhand (palm-down) grip. Right: Underhand (palm-up) grip.

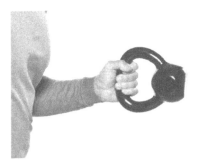

Thumb-up grip.

grip is often used when performing swings.

Underhand (Palm Up): Grab the handle from beneath (with your palm up). This grip is often used in arm curl movements.

Thumb Up: Grab the handle with an overhand grip then rotate the hand so the thumb is up. For people with shoulder concerns, this grip is more comfortable when performing overhead presses.

Side by Side (Double Hand): Place your hands side by side on top of the handle with an overhand (palm-down) grip. This grip is often used when doing upright rowing motions, heavy deadlifts, swings or as a start grip

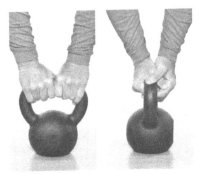

Left: Side-by-side (double-hand) grip. Right: Hand-over/on-hand grip.

for grab-and-release moves. You can also try a side-by-side grip with palms facing each other.

Hand over/on Hand: Place one hand on top of the handle and then the other hand on top of that hand. This grip is often used for heavy swings and grab-and-release moves. It's also preferred by those with hand issues.

Rack Position: The rack position is where the kettlebell move either ends or begins. In the rack position, the kettlebell rests against the outside of your forearm, with your elbow as close to your ribs as possible. The handle of the bell should be slightly above the belly of the kettlebell. To get to rack position, you can perform a clean or, if the kettlebell is light, an arm curl.

The Clean (page 89) is the hallmark move of kettlebell training. This move is much like what's seen in Olympic lifting, except in kettlebell training it's one-handed in most cases. This is a ballistic move used to get a heavy kettlebell to the rack position.

Overhead Lockout Position: The top position of an overhead press or a snatch is often referred to as the "lockout." The hand is turned slightly toward the body and is directly over the shoulder; the kettlebell handle rests diagonally across the palm and the fingers are often just slightly bent to hold on to the handle.

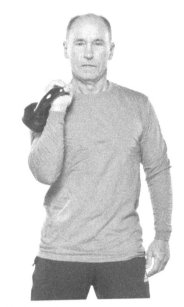

Rack position

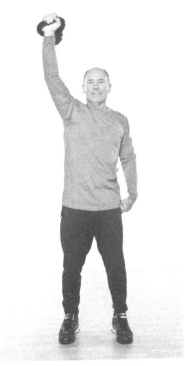

Overhead lockout position

part 2

the

programs

how to use this book

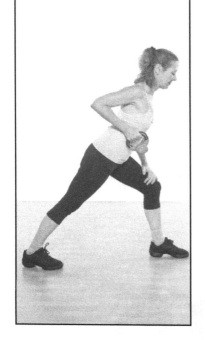

Kettlebells for 50+ is composed of exercises for everyone, from beginners to weekend warriors to longtime athletes. These exercises can complement an existing fitness program or serve as the components to a standalone routine. Kettlebell training can be anything you need it to be, from a fun and exciting method for staying in shape to an intense workout to build power and great levels of strength.

This section features several routines, from general conditioning to power-building to sport-specific. They can be used as standalone workouts or done for a few weeks when you're bored of your usual program. All exercises, complete with instructions and photographs, appear in Part 3 and are organized in order from foundational to more complex. These exercises will improve muscular strength and endurance and foster better neuromuscular coordination than any selectorized weight-machine workout.

Note that though you may choose to follow one of these routines, you can still modify the workout as necessary. Some days you might feel strong and other days weak. Go with what your body tells you. It's better to do a little bit of anything than a lot of nothing. Enjoy the fluidity of movement and go with the flow of the kettlebell. Exercise for yourself! My goal is for you to become internally motivated to engage in the kettlebell exercise rather than feel like you have to exercise.

If you choose a sport-specific workout, it's assumed you know not to overtrain. Consider doing the kettlebell series as an adjunct to your existing routine or as an off-season conditioning program. Train to play, not the other way around!

Many of my clients like the concept of cross-training, where you perform your regular workout (say, Monday and Wednesday) and, for a change of venue, do a kettlebell workout on Friday along with push-ups, pull-ups and dips. The routines are by no means absolute—feel free to adapt them as you see fit. If you have an existing fitness program, select some kettlebell exercises and integrate them into your existing routine. Switching different kettlebell moves in and out of your workout every few weeks keeps your exercise regimen fresh and prevents it from becoming stale. Making your routine a living document will keep kettlebell training fun and innovative! Consider the exercises in Part 3 as a guideline and mix and match different exercises to challenge your muscles or accommodate your limitations. For more information about designing your own program, turn to page 29.

If you haven't yet selected the right kettlebell for you, read the tips on page 20. Depending on your goals, you may need one on the lighter side and one on the heavier side. In general, for all moves, you should start with a light kettlebell and see how your body responds while you learn the movements and place them in your muscle memory. Only increase kettlebell weight or progress to more advanced exercises after you've mastered the basic exercises.

If you experience any discomfort, back off on the number of reps you perform, reduce the load or ask someone to observe you as you perform the movement so that they can give you feedback to help you make corrections.

Common Terms

It may be helpful to familiarize yourself with common fitness terminology and concepts.

Cross-training: A method of training in which you engage in a variety of training methods (e.g., lift weights at the gym on Monday and Wednesday, do a kettlebell workout at home on Friday).

Flexibility: The range of motion around a joint. An example is being able to move freely and comfortably through a complete range of motion.

Muscular endurance: The ability of a muscle to contract for a prolonged period of time.

Muscular strength: The amount of weight/force a muscle can exert.

When learning any new exercise, especially with kettlebells, it's best to focus on form first rather than worry about how much you can lift or how quickly you can do it. Learn to "feel the move" and place the move into muscle memory. An example of this is the Upright Row (page 65). Most people don't pay attention to retracting/squeezing their shoulder blades throughout the movement or keeping their back in a neutral position (i.e., not allowing their back to round)— they're thinking about how much weight they can lift, which shouldn't be the goal of this or any exercise. For a muscle to memorize a move, you must do the movement over and over until muscle memory has occurred. Once you've learned the move, you can then introduce a heavier load.

Overload principle training: When you slowly load the muscles beyond normal capacity to promote muscular strength and/or endurance.

Overtraining: When a training routine exceeds the person's capabilities, creating a deleterious outcome to the trainee.

Periodization: A systematic approach of changing your training routine at a regularly scheduled interval.

Power: A combination of speed and strength applied over a short period of time.

Plyometrics: Exercises (usually involving hopping and jumping)

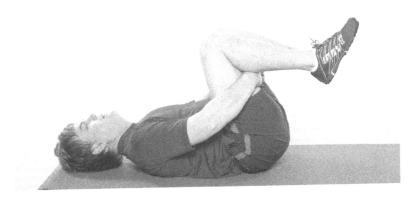

that maximize the stretch reflex to teach muscles to produce maximum force.

Progression: The process of changing the challenges placed upon the body (usually intensity, volume and frequency) to stimulate desired gains.

Progressive resistance exercise: Commonly referred to as strength training, where you systematically increase the load to challenge a muscle as it gets stronger.

Recovery/Rest: The rest interval placed between sets or days to allow the muscles to recover from an exercise or a workout.

Rep: The number of times you perform a movement.

Set: The grouping of reps (e.g., 2 sets of 3 reps would require you to do a move 3 times, rest and do the move 3 more times).

Specificity of training: Matching your physical training program to your specific demands.

Superset: The execution of two exercises with no rest until at least two superset exercises are completed (e.g., Gunslinger Curl and Arm Curl). Another approach could be to perform opposing muscle group exercises, such as Gunslinger Curl followed immediately by a Bent-Over Triceps Extension. Supersets are often used in hypertrophy (muscle cell enlargement).

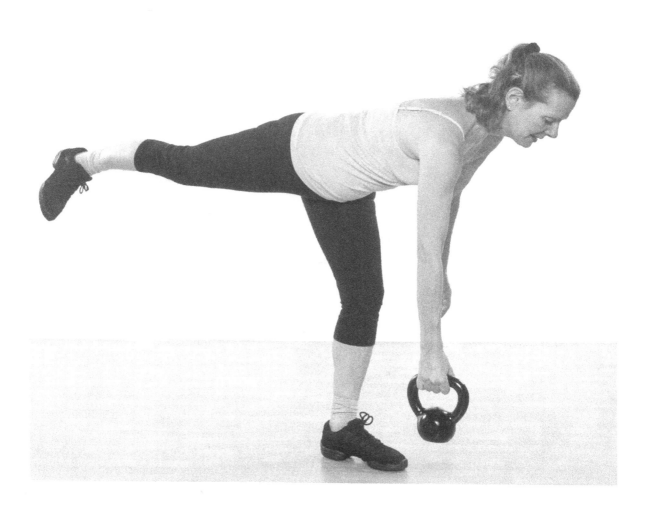

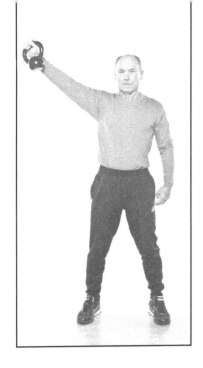

designing your own workout

A well-designed exercise program will help you function better in activities of daily living as well as in sports. The beauty of a kettlebell is that it can be used to meet a number of fitness goals. If the routines on pages 32–46 aren't quite what you're looking for, you can personalize your own workout.

An important concept in fitness training today is "functional training." The philosophy behind this is to train the muscles to "function" in a variety of ways that mimic the movements engaged in daily living or when participating in a sport. Unfortunately, today we're finding that many older adults can't perform "normal" functional activities of daily life. It's not uncommon to find a 65-year-old having a hard time getting up easily from the floor because their leg strength has deteriorated. The term *sarcopenia* is what scientists call atrophy caused by a sedentary lifestyle. More simply put: Move it or lose it!

Functional training is usually based on a progression of movements, graduated from simple to complex and from slow to fast. Functional training routines generally begin with isolation-type exercises that work one or two muscles around a single joint, working up to compound movements, such as on page 77. This principle applies whether you're a world-class athlete, post-rehab person or baby boomer. *Kettlebells for 50+* takes the same approach.

When you design a functional fitness program using kettlebells, every effort should be placed on making the program real. Include movements that have practical applications, fostering sound postural alignment and always following a good biomechanical pattern; maintain a proper base of support, improve flexibility and joint mobility and balance strength vs. dynamic stability. In addition, coordinate proper sequencing of movement with proper motor control.

A sound, functional, progressive-resistance kettlebell exercise program should have a balance between progressions of strength, speed, agility and power. A balanced program should also address eccentric vs. concentric moves and closed-kinetic-chain and open-kinetic-chain exercises. Let's use the Sumo Squat (page 49) to illustrate eccentric vs. concentric movements: Lifting the kettlebell up is the concentric portion of the movement, while lowering the kettlebell to the floor is the eccentric portion. The Lunge (page 60) is an example of a closed-kinetic-chain exercise for the legs when the feet are planted on the floor. The basic arm curl (page 77) is a common example of an open-kinetic-chain exercise. For a comprehensive exercise program, be sure to include some cardiovascular exercises such as walking, biking and swimming.

The key to a successful kettlebell experience is knowing how and when to incorporate the above training principles into your routine. To prevent an injury, understand how to incorporate intensity, duration, frequency and mode in a safe and sane manner. You have two options: Train hard and make improvements quickly but get hurt and quit; or train smart, lessen your risk of getting injured and stay motivated to continue. Don't focus on being better than someone else. Instead, focus on being healthier and better tomorrow. Slow and steady wins the fitness race.

Here are several elements you should include in your individualized kettlebell workout: a warm-up, exercises that address your goals, a cool-down/stretch. Other elements that should be included in your overall fitness routine are regular 20- to 30-minute bouts of comfortably paced aerobic exercise most days of the week, as well as proper nutrition.

Warming Up

Since exercising with a kettlebell is a total-body exercise, it's recommended that you perform an active thermal warm-up, perhaps by going for a light jog for 5–10 minutes, jogging/jumping in place, skipping rope or riding a stationary bike. You can also check out the warm-up suggestions on pages 92–100. The purpose of the warm-up is to enhance core temperature and ready the muscles and joints for an exercise session. Don't confuse warming up and stretching. Warming up increases the temperature of the muscles, much like warming up the old '57 Chevy before a drive. Stretching is a passive activity.

Once your body is warmed up, perform your favorite full-body kettlebell exercises at a slow speed or with a light weight to prepare your body for the more engaging movements. This warm-up concept is the same as when you prepare for a round of tennis by hitting the ball back and forth before playing the actual game. Once your body is warmed up, you can start your workout. Failure to adequately warm up can set you up for an injury. Other warm-up approaches

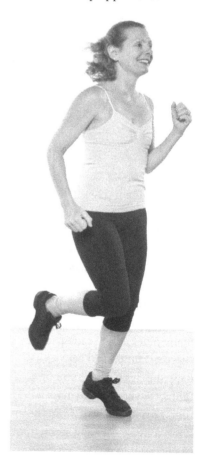

involve sitting in a sauna, warm shower or bath, or even putting a heat pack on a stubborn body part (shoulder, back).

Training for Your Goal

An effective kettlebell program for a 50+ person needs to be unique to the individual. Pick moves that best meet your particular needs and mood. As stated earlier in the book, kettlebell training for 50+ folks is not about a prescriptive routine designed for you but rather a routine designed by you and for you. You're the captain of your fitness ship! Adapt and modify your kettlebell program by tweaking each session. Include exercises that allow you to move in manners that respect your 50+ frame and are enjoyable to you without causing you any discomfort.

Keep in mind that age-related muscle loss (sarcopenia) and bone loss (osteoporosis) are becoming major health concerns for 50+ folks. Therefore, improving muscle mass needs to be a goal for the 50+ person who desires to grow well, not old.

Kettlebells are also an excellent tool to foster improved sports performance. To effectively use kettlebells to improve performance, learn to understand the demands and skills of your sport—this is the key. A sport may even have several positions that require different skills. When designing this kind of workout, consider the following:

- What are the physical requirements of your sport (e.g., strength, power, flexibility, agility, speed, quickness, coordination)?
- Does your sport rely on raw athletic traits or precision?
- Does your sport require greater upper body strength or leg strength?

The "FITT" concept is an excellent model to follow when designing your special program.

F stands for **Frequency**, or the number of times something is done. To obtain optimal results, you should perform your kettlebell workout 1–2 times a week. The more frequently you can exercise, the better the results.

I stands for **Intensity**, or how heavy a weight you lift. The intensity is determined by your goals. When building strength, go heavy and do the move 6–8 times. For general fitness, aim for 10 times. As you become more fit, increase the intensity.

T stands for **Time**, or the length/duration of each training session. To gain physical results, you should train long enough that mild muscle fatigue occurs, then rest long enough to feel refreshed (usually after a 30-second rest). "Time" and "reps" are interchangeable terms. A time/rep is dependent on the load you're doing—10 rep/times is a good rule of thumb for general fitness. As you become more fit, increase the time on task and reduce recovery time.

T stands for **Type**, or the mode of activity that you perform to produce the desired results. In this case it's kettlebells.

Cooling Down & Stretching

After you're done with your kettlebell workout, spend 5–10 minutes stretching the major joints and muscles of the body, such as shoulders, hamstrings, calves, back, neck and hands. Stretches start on page 101. If you have a problem area, spend extra time at that location and consider using ice on the area. Stretching after an exercise session, while the muscles are warm and more receptive, is ideal. Post-exercise stretching helps maintain mobility of the joints. As a person gets older, a daily dose of flexibility works wonders in warding off stiffness.

introduction to kettlebells

This general-fitness kettlebell workout is geared toward those who are new to lifting weights or kettlebell training. Perform all motions without a kettlebell several times until you're familiar with the motions and how your body reacts to them. Then practice gripping the kettlebell. Start with a kettlebell weight that you can lift at least 5 times then progress to 15 reps.

Perform this program for at least 2 weeks before progressing to the next level. If you display any discomfort, back off or eliminate any exercise that produces that discomfort. Always perform a thermal warm-up for at least 10 minutes to prepare your body for exercise. Post-workout stretches have been included to facilitate flexibility and reduce injury.

INTRODUCTION TO KETTLEBELLS

Warm up for at least 10 minutes. See pages 92–100 for suggestions.

EXERCISE	SETS	REP/TIME	REST
Double-Bell Squat *p. 51*	1	5–10	30 sec
Bodyweight Deadlift *p. 96*	1	5–10	30 sec
Overhead Press *p. 63*	1	5–10	30 sec
Sword Fighter *p. 69*	1	5–10	30 sec
Picture Frame *p. 103*	1	30 sec	30 sec
Soup Can Pour *p. 108*	1	30 sec	30 sec
Double Knee to Chest *p. 116*	1	30 sec	30 sec

level 1

How do you know when you're ready to start this level? If the Introduction to Kettlebells workout seems too easy, then you're ready. However, if you're experiencing some soreness or awkwardness with the movements, don't progress until you're more comfortable.

Always perform a thermal warm-up for at least 5 minutes to prepare your body for the workout. Then try out all kettlebell motions without a kettlebell until you're familiar with the movements. After your kettlebell routine perform the post-workout stretches that have been included to facilitate flexibility and reduce injury. In this program, start to challenge yourself by increasing the load or extending the time you perform the movements.

LEVEL 1

Warm up for at least 10 minutes. See pages 92–100 for suggestions.

EXERCISE	SETS	REP/TIME	REST
Double-Bell Squat *p. 51*	1–2	5–15	30 sec
Deadlift *p. 57*	1–2	5–15	30 sec
Bent-Over Row *p. 67*	1–2	5–15	30 sec
Curl-Up *p. 73*	1–2	5–15	30 sec
Gunslinger Curl *p. 81*	1–2	5–15	30 sec
Picture Frame *p. 103*	1	30 sec	--
Soup Can Pour *p. 108*	1	30 sec	--
Double Wood Chop *p. 107*	1	30 sec	--
Wrist Stretch *p. 120*	1	30 sec	--
Wrist Circles *p. 121*	1	30 sec	--

By the time you move to this level, you should feel confident with the kettlebell movements. Your level of fitness should also be increasing and you should be ready to start challenging yourself. Only you will know when you're ready. If you overdo it, your body will tell you; back off a little or downsize some of the exercises in this workout to best match your current level. Treat this fitness routine as a living document that can be amended as needed. Nothing is written in stone.

Always perform a thermal warm-up for at least 5 minutes to prepare your body for the workout. Then try out all kettlebell motions with a lighter kettlebell until you're familiar with the movements. Finally, challenge yourself by pushing up the reps or load. Since you'll be including a second set, consider doing the first set lighter with more reps and the second set heavier with less reps. Post-workout stretches have been included to facilitate flexibility and reduce injury.

LEVEL 2

Warm up for at least 10 minutes. See pages 92–100 for suggestions.

EXERCISE	SETS	REP/TIME	REST
Double-Bell Squat *p. 51*	2	5–15	30 sec
Side-Step Squat *p. 54*	2	5–15	30 sec
Overhead Press *p. 63*	2	5–15	30 sec
Bent-Over Row *p. 67*	2	5–15	30 sec
Bent-Over Triceps Extension *p. 68*	2	5–15	30 sec
Double-Bell Kneeling Get-Up *p. 74*	2	5–15	30 sec
Curl-Up *p. 73*	2	5–15	30 sec
Plank *p. 99*	2	1 min max	30 sec
Lateral Arm Raise & Squat *p. 79*	2	5–15	30 sec
Calf Stretch *p. 112*	2	30 sec	15 sec
Zipper *p. 110*	2	30 sec	15 sec
V Stretch *p. 115*	2	30 sec	15 sec
Mad Cat *p. 113*	2	30 sec	15 sec

level 3

If Level 2 seems too easy and you feel no discomfort, you're ready to try Level 3. Your body will tell you when to proceed and when to back off. If some portions of this workout are too difficult, you can keep some of your favorites from Level 2 if you wish.

In this workout, the rest time has been shortened and you should be pushing to increase the load. Consider challenging yourself by progressively increasing the load and reps. This workout is really the beginning of a solid fitness routine. Treat it as a living document that can be amended as needed. Nothing is written in stone.

Always perform a thermal warm-up for at least 5 minutes to prepare your body for the workout. Then try out all kettlebell motions with a lighter kettlebell until you're familiar with the movements. Since you'll be including a second set, consider doing the first set lighter with more reps and the second set heavier with less reps. The third set should lie somewhere in between. Post-workout stretches have been included to facilitate flexibility and reduce injury.

LEVEL 3

Warm up for at least 10 minutes. See pages 92–100 for suggestions.

EXERCISE	SETS	REP/TIME	REST
Single-Bell Squat p. 50	3	5–15	15 sec
Deadlift p. 57	3	5–15	15 sec
Lunge p. 60	3	5–15	15 sec
Lunge with Overhead Lockout p. 62	3	5–15	15 sec
Plank Rotation with Arm Extension p. 72	3	5–15	15 sec
Rocking Horse p. 76	3	5–15	15 sec
Double-Bell Kneeling Get-Up p. 74	3	5–15	15 sec
Arm Curl & Leg Curl p. 77	3	5–15	15 sec
Diagonal Knee to Chest p. 117	2	30 sec	10 sec
Side-to-Side Neck Stretch p. 101	2	30 sec	10 sec
Neck Half-Circles p. 102	2	30 sec	10 sec
Butterfly p. 114	2	30 sec	10 sec
Wrist Stretch p. 120	2	30 sec	10 sec
Wrist Circles p. 121	2	30 sec	10 sec

powerhouse

This advanced-level workout, designed to foster greater levels of power, is for elite 50+ athletes who are highly trained and can or have performed heavy resistance training in the past. Your doctor has cleared you in the past for high-intensity training—your blood pressure is within acceptable limits and you're pain-free.

This workout can be hard on joints and should only be done 1–2 times a week for no more than 4 weeks. After you've performed this workout for 4 weeks, back off for a period. This routine will push you to your limits—don't overdo it. Most people won't do this routine nor need to. Treat this routine as a living document that can be amended as needed. Nothing is written in stone.

Always perform a thermal warm-up for at least 10 minutes to prepare your body for the workout. Note that since this workout encourages heavy lifting, greater recovery time between sets and fewer reps are necessary. Since you'll be including a second set, consider doing the first set lighter with more reps and the second set heavier with less reps. The third set should lie somewhere in between. Post-workout stretches have been included to facilitate flexibility and reduce injury.

POWERHOUSE

Warm up for at least 10 minutes. See pages 92–100 for suggestions.

EXERCISE	SETS	REP/TIME	REST
Double-Bell Squat *p. 51*	1–3	3–5	60 sec
Lunge with Overhead Lockout *p. 62*	1–3	3–5	60 sec
Double-Bell Overhead Press *p. 63*	1–3	3–5	60 sec
Bent-Over Row *p. 67*	1–3	3–5	60 sec
Double-Bell Kneeling Get-Up & Press *p. 75*	1–3	3–5	60 sec
V Stretch *p. 115*	1–3	30–60 sec	30 sec
Quad Stretch *p. 111*	1–3	30–60 sec	30 sec
Calf Stretch *p. 112*	1–3	30–60 sec	30 sec
Wrist Stretch *p. 120*	1–3	30–60 sec	30 sec
Wrist Circles *p. 121*	1–3	30–60 sec	30 sec
Zipper *p. 110*	1–3	30–60 sec	30 sec

This routine is designed for highly motivated and fit individuals who are highly trained and can or have performed heavy resistance training in the past. Your doctor has cleared you in the past for high-intensity training—your blood pressure is within acceptable limits and you're pain-free. Don't perform this routine unless you're in super shape and are prepared for a little muscle soreness.

Since it includes swings and releases, this workout requires good hand-eye coordination. It should only be done 1–2 times a week for no more than 4 weeks. After you've performed this workout for 4 weeks, back off for a period. Treat this routine as a living document that can be amended as needed. Nothing is written in stone.

Always perform a thermal warm-up for at least 10 minutes to prepare your body for the workout. Since you'll be including a second set, consider doing the first set lighter with more reps and the second set heavier with less reps. The third set should lie somewhere in between. If you're super-fit, try 4 sets. Post-workout stretches have been included to facilitate flexibility and reduce injury.

SUPER-ADVANCED FITNESS AND COORDINATION

Warm up for at least 10 minutes. See pages 92–100 for suggestions.

EXERCISE	SETS	REP/TIME	REST
Sword Fighter *p. 69*	2–3	8–15	20 sec
Alternating Overhead Press *p. 64*	2–3	8–15	20 sec
Plank Row Rotation *p. 71*	2–3	8–15	20 sec
Rocking Horse with Press *p. 76*	2–3	8–15	20 sec
Kneeling Get-Up & Press *p. 75*	2–3	8–15	20 sec
Lateral Arm Raise & Squat *p. 79*	2–3	8–15	20 sec
Figure 8 *p. 86*	2–3	8–15	20 sec
Double-Arm Swing *p. 83*	2–3	8–15	20 sec
Single-Arm Swing *p. 85*	2–3	8–15	20 sec
Alternating Swing & Catch *p. 88*	2–3	8–15	20 sec
Piriformis Stretch *p. 119*	2	45 sec	20 sec
Pec Stretch #1 *p. 104*	2	45 sec	20 sec
Pec Stretch #2 *p. 105*	2	45 sec	20 sec
Rotator Cuff *p. 109*	2	45 sec	20 sec
V Stretch *p. 115*	2	45 sec	20 sec
Butterfly *p. 114*	2	45 sec	20 sec
Calf Stretch *p. 112*	2	45 sec	20 sec
Mad Cat *p. 113*	2	45 sec	20 sec
Wrist Stretch *p. 120*	2	45 sec	20 sec
Wrist Circles *p. 121*	2	45 sec	20 sec

baseball/softball

This hurry-up-and-wait sport has a great deal of standing or sitting around and then calls upon its players to quickly react to a situation or ball. A middle infielder will have a different workout than a catcher or an outfielder so adapt this routine to the specific needs of your position. Speak to your coach about the specific requirements of your position. As you become more fit, decrease the recovery time and increase the load. The intensity of your training depends on your level of play. If you're a tournament player, use this routine to prepare yourself for the season.

BASEBALL/SOFTBALL

Warm up for at least 10 minutes. See pages 92–100 for suggestions.

EXERCISE	SETS	REP/TIME	REST
Forward Lunge *p. 60*	1–2	10–15	30 sec
Backward Lunge *p. 60*	1–2	10–15	30 sec
Side-Step Squat *p. 54*	1–2	10–15	30 sec
Sword Fighter *p. 69*	1–2	10–15	30 sec
Bent-Over Row *p. 67*	1–2	10–15	30 sec
Plank Row Rotation *p. 71*	1–2	10–15	30 sec
Double-Bell Kneeling Get-Up *p. 74*	1–2	10–15	30 sec
Curl-Up *p. 73*	1–2	10–15	30 sec
Figure 8 *p. 86*	1–2	10–15	30 sec
Alternating Swing & Catch *p. 88*	1–2	10–15	30 sec
Mad Cat *p. 113*	1–2	60 sec	30 sec
Wrist Stretch *p. 120*	1–2	60 sec	30 sec
Wrist Circles *p. 121*	1–2	60 sec	30 sec
Butterfly *p. 114*	1–2	60 sec	30 sec
Rotator Cuff *p. 109*	1–2	60 sec	30 sec
Soup Can Pour *p. 108*	1–2	60 sec	30 sec
Picture Frame *p. 103*	1–2	60 sec	30 sec
Zipper *p. 110*	1–2	60 sec	30 sec

basketball

Basketball requires an excellent aerobic baseline to accommodate bouts of explosive speed and jumps. If you're practicing and playing a couple of games a week, you might just do this workout in the off-season to reduce your risk of overtraining or use it as a pre-season conditioning routine. Train to play, not the other way around! As you become more fit, decrease rest time.

BASKETBALL

Warm up for at least 10 minutes. See pages 92–100 for suggestions.

EXERCISE	SETS	REP/TIME	REST
Single-Bell Racked Squat p. 52	2–3	10–15	15–30 sec
Side-Step Squat p. 54	2–3	10–15	15–30 sec
Bodyweight Deadlift p. 96	2–3	10–15	30 sec
Plank Row p. 70	2	10–15	15–30 sec
Gunslinger Curl p. 81	2	10–15	15–30 sec
Double-Arm Swing p. 83	2	10–15	15–30 sec
V Stretch p. 115	2	60 sec	10 sec
Piriformis Stretch p. 119	2	60 sec	10 sec
Double Knee to Chest p. 116	2	60 sec	10 sec
Pec Stretch #1 p. 104	2	60 sec	15–30 sec
Pec Stretch #2 p. 105	2	60 sec	15–30 sec
Double Wood Chop p. 107	2	60 sec	15–30 sec
Quad Stretch p. 111	2	60 sec	30 sec
Side-to-Side Neck Stretch p. 101	2	60 sec	30 sec
Neck Half-Circles p. 102	2	60 sec	30 sec
Butterfly p. 114	2	60 sec	30 sec

golf

When designing a golf program, check with your golf pro to see which kettlebell moves best serve your particular needs and think about which muscles are involved in golf. Since golf is an asymmetrical sport, you'll need to make sure to train both sides in order to balance out your body. The level of your training is dependent on you—the recreational player has a different agenda than a tournament player. Be careful with low back moves since many golfers have a bad back. My recommendation is to perform kettlebell workouts in the off-season.

GOLF

Warm up for at least 10 minutes. See pages 92–100 for suggestions.

EXERCISE	SETS	REP/TIME	REST
Bodyweight Deadlift *p. 96*	1–2	8–10	30 sec
Side-Step Squat *p. 54*	1–2	8–10	30 sec
Plank Row Rotation *p. 71*	1–2	8–10	30 sec
Curl-Up *p. 73*	1–2	8–10	30 sec
One-Legged Deadlift *p. 58*	1–2	8–10	30 sec
Single-Bell Squat *p. 50*	1–2	8–10	30 sec
Side-to-Side Neck Stretch *p. 101*	1–2	30 sec	30 sec
Double Knee to Chest *p. 116*	1–2	30 sec	30 sec
Pec Stretch #2 *p. 105*	1–2	30 sec	30 sec
Piriformis Stretch *p. 119*	1–2	30 sec	30 sec
Calf Stretch *p. 112*	1–2	30 sec	30 sec
Double Wood Chop *p. 107*	1–2	30 sec	30 sec

kayaking

Kayaking can be a recreational hobby done paddling around a lagoon or can be an intense sport when performed in rivers or the open seas. Kayaking demands upper-body endurance along with strength and power to place the kayak on top of the car or to carry it down to the beach. Some level of lower-body strength is needed as well, not to mention excellent core stability. Kayaking requires strength and endurance on both sides of the body. The intensity of your kettlebell program is dependent on the level of fitness you need. It's also wise to add an aerobic component to your routine.

KAYAKING

Warm up for at least 10 minutes. See pages 92–100 for suggestions.

EXERCISE	SETS	REP/TIME	REST
Sumo Squat *p. 49*	2	8–10	60 sec
Single-Bell Squat *p. 50*	2	8–10	60 sec
Single-Bell Racked Squat *p. 52*	2	8–10	60 sec
Racked Lunge *p. 61*	2	10–15	30 sec
Overhead Press *p. 63*	2	10–15	30 sec
Upright Row *p. 65*	2	10–15	30 sec
Bent-Over Row *p. 67*	3	10–15	30 sec
Sword Fighter *p. 69*	3	10–15	30 sec
Plank Row *p. 70*	3	30 sec	30 sec
Curl-Up *p. 73*	3	60 sec	30 sec
Lateral Arm Raise & Squat *p. 79*	3	10–15	30 sec
Double-Arm Swing *p. 83*	1	8–10	60 sec
Single-Arm Swing *p. 85*	2	8–10	60 sec
Clean & Press *p. 90*	1	6-8	--
Bodyweight Lunge *p. 95*	1	30 sec	--
Bodyweight Deadlift *p. 96*	1	30 sec	--
Arm Swing with Neck Turn *p. 97*	1	60 sec	--
Neck Half-Circles *p. 102*	1	30 sec	--
Pec Stretch #1 *p. 104*	1	30 sec	--

skiing

Downhill skiing can be a fun recreational hobby done on the bunny slopes or an extreme sport that tackles the black diamonds of the mountains. The intensity of your kettlebell routine is dependent upon your expectations. The ability to enjoy a full day of skiing is dependent on the strength and endurance of your legs and core.

SKIING

Warm up for at least 10 minutes. See pages 92–100 for suggestions.

EXERCISE	SETS	REP/TIME	REST
Sumo Squat p. 49	3	10–15	60 sec
Side-Step Squat p. 54	3	10–15	60 sec
Lunge p. 60	3	10–15	60 sec
Sword Fighter p. 69	2	8–10	30 sec
Plank Row p. 70	2	5-7	60 sec
Curl-Up p. 73	2	10–15	60 sec
Double-Bell Kneeling Get-Up p. 74	2	10–15	30 sec
Arm Curl & Leg Curl p. 77	2	8–10	30 sec
Double-Arm Swing p. 83	2	10–15	30 sec
Jumping Jacks p. 92	1	60 sec	--
Knee Lift p. 93	1	2 min	--
Bodyweight Squat p. 94	1	30 sec	--
Bodyweight Lunge p. 95	1	30 sec	--
Bodyweight Deadlift p. 96	1	10	--
Plank p. 99	2	30 sec	--
Quad Stretch p. 111	2	30 sec	15 sec
Butterfly p. 114	2	30 sec	15 sec
Calf Stretch p. 112	2	30 sec	15 sec

soccer

This sport requires cardiovascular endurance, muscular endurance, agility and explosive speed, among other physical qualities. As you're well aware, each position has its own subset of physical requirements so design the kettlebell workout to best suit your positional needs. Speak with your coach as to how best to include kettlebells in your existing training routine. If you're playing soccer several times a week and playing on the weekends, this kettlebell workout is best done in the off-season to avoid overtraining injuries. It can be performed as a pre-season conditioning program to complement your existing programs. As your fitness increases, decrease recovery time and increase reps and intensity.

SOCCER

Warm up for at least 10 minutes. See pages 92–100 for suggestions.

EXERCISE	SETS	REP/TIME	REST
Bodyweight Deadlift p. 96	2	8–10	20 sec
Side-Step Squat p. 54	2	8–10	20 sec
Forward Lunge p. 60	2	8–10	20 sec
Backward Lunge p. 60	2	8–10	20 sec
Plank Row p. 70	2	8–10	20 sec
Plank Row Rotation p. 71	2	8–10	20 sec
Plank Rotation with Arm Extension p. 72	2	8–10	20 sec
Double-Bell Kneeling Get-Up p. 74	2	8–10	20 sec
Arm Curl & Leg Curl p. 77	2	8–10	20 sec
Double-Arm Swing (light) p. 83	2	8–10	20 sec
Double Knee to Chest p. 116	2	60 sec	10 sec
Diagonal Knee to Chest p. 117	2	60 sec	10 sec
V Stretch p. 115	2	60 sec	10 sec
Butterfly p. 114	2	60 sec	10 sec
Side-to-Side Neck Stretch p. 101	2	60 sec	10 sec

surfing

Surfing can be a fun recreational hobby done in the lapping waves of Honolulu or can be an intense sport done in major waves in chilly water. Surfing requires upper-body endurance to paddle out to the waves and explosive power to stand up quickly. It also demands excellent balance and agility. The intensity of your kettlebell routine should be done according to your intentions.

SURFING

Warm up for at least 10 minutes. See pages 92–100 for suggestions.

EXERCISE	SETS	REP/TIME	REST
Lunge with Overhead Lockout *p. 62*	2	10–15	30 sec
Bent-Over Triceps Extension *p. 68*	3	10–15	30 sec
Sword Fighter *p. 69*	3	10–15	30 sec
Plank Row Rotation *p. 71*	2	5–10	30 sec
Kneeling Get-Up & Press *p. 75*	3	10–15	30 sec
Double Swing *p. 83*	3	10–15	30 sec
Single-Arm Swing *p. 85*	3	10–15	30 sec
Figure 8 *p. 86*	2	5–10	60 sec
Alternating Swing & Catch *p. 88*	3	10–15	30 sec
Arm Swings with Neck Turn *p. 97*	1	45 sec	--
Pec Stretch #2 *p. 105*	2	30 sec	15 sec
Double Wood Chop *p. 107*	2	45 sec	15 sec
Soup Can Pour *p. 108*	1	10–15	--
Rotator Cuff *p. 109*	1	10–15	--
Mad Cat *p. 113*	1	10–15	--

swimming

Swimming is an excellent method to develop overall fitness. However, since it's not weight bearing, all swimmers should do some level of weight training. Therefore, a regular dose of kettlebell training 2–3 times week is an excellent idea. Swimming involves many types of strokes, from freestyle to butterfly, so if you're a competitive swimmer, speak with your coach about what the most important muscles are for you. Keep in mind that many swimmers have shoulder issues so be careful to not overdo the shoulder motions or use excessively heavy kettlebells.

SWIMMING

Warm up for at least 10 minutes. See pages 92–100 for suggestions.

EXERCISE	SETS	REP/TIME	REST
Lunge *p. 60*	2	10–15	30 sec
Upright Row *p. 65*	2	10–15	30 sec
Bent-Over Triceps Extension *p. 68*	2	10–15	30 sec
Sword Fighter *p. 69*	3	10–15	30 sec
Kneeling Get-Up & Press *p. 75*	2	8–10	30 sec
Arm Curl & Leg Curl *p. 77*	2	8–10	30 sec
Overhead Press & Squat *p. 80*	2	8–10	30 sec
Gunslinger Curl *p. 81*	2	8–10	30 sec
Double-Arm Swing *p. 83*	3	10–15	30 sec
Bodyweight Squat *p. 94*	2	10–15	30 sec
Bodyweight Lunge *p. 95*	1	10–15	--
Arm Circles *p. 98*	1	10–15	--
Plank *p. 99*	2	30 sec	15 sec
Pec Stretch #2 *p. 105*	2	30 sec	15 sec
Double Wood Chop *p. 107*	1	60 sec	15 sec
Soup Can Pour *p. 108*	1	10	--
Rotator Cuff *p. 109*	1	10	--
Zipper *p. 110*	2	30 sec	15 sec
Mad Cat *p. 113*	1	10	15 sec

tennis

Tennis is a sport that can be played well into later life and is played at all levels. As you know, tennis involves quick starts and stops and prolonged matches. If you're not doing two-handed backhands, it can be a somewhat one-sided sport, which means upper body imbalances. Thus your kettlebell routine should be designed for your level of play and fitness level. Ask your tennis pro to review your workout to match your level of play. Try to design one that equalizes the development on both sides of the body. This kettlebell workout should complement your existing training schedule. Use caution when doing kettlebell moves that include the knee and shoulders. Since the shoulder joint in 50+ tennis players is already at risk for injury, consider my other book *Healthy Shoulder Handbook*, also published by Ulysses Press.

TENNIS

Warm up for at least 10 minutes. See pages 92–100 for suggestions.

EXERCISE	SETS	REP/TIME	REST
Side-Step Squat *p. 54*	2	10–15	30–45 sec
Overhead Press *p. 63*	2	10–15	30–45 sec
Sword Fighter *p. 69*	2	10–15	30 sec
Plank Row Rotation *p. 71*	2	10–15	45 sec
Curl-Up *p. 73*	2	10–15	30 sec
Gunslinger Curl *p. 81*	2	10–15	30 sec
Double-Arm Swing *p. 83*	2	10–15	45 sec
Figure 8 *p. 86*	2	10–15	30 sec
Mad Cat *p. 113*	2	45 sec	10 sec
Wrist Stretch *p. 120*	2	45 sec	10 sec
Wrist Circles *p. 121*	2	45 sec	10 sec
Quad Stretch *p. 111*	2	45 sec	20 sec
Butterfly *p. 114*	2	45 sec	30 sec
Rotator Cuff *p. 109*	2	45 sec	30 sec
Soup Can Pour *p. 108*	2	45 sec	30 sec
Double Wood Chop *p. 107*	2	45 sec	20 sec
Zipper *p. 110*	2	45 sec	30 sec
Piriformis Stretch *p. 119*	2	45 sec	30 sec
Side-to-Side Neck Stretch *p. 101*	2	45 sec	30 sec

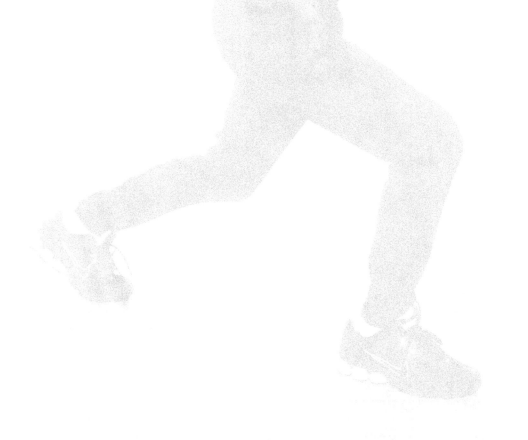

part 3

the
exercises

squat series

The squat series is designed to enhance the power and strength of the legs as well as tone the torso. The legs are the foundation of independence for 50+ folks. For all squats, keep your back in neutral position, your head up, and your legs a comfortable distance apart. Engage your core, and try to keep your heels down. Lower yourself down until your thighs are parallel with the floor. Make sure your knees point in the same direction as your feet throughout the movement; to protect your knees, don't allow them to extend past your toes. As you get stronger, you may move on to heavier bells.

If you need to modify any of these squats, feel free to either squat into a chair or place the kettlebell on a table or block so you don't need to lower yourself down as much.

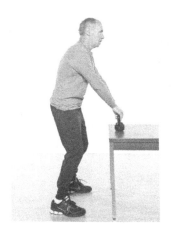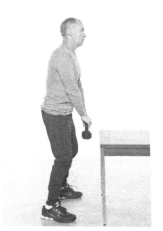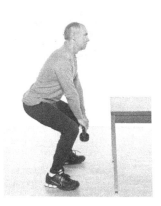

Table modification

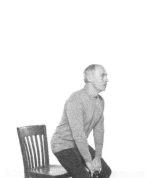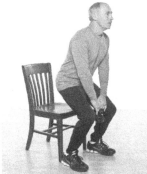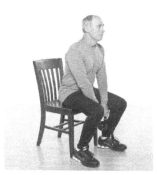

Chair modification

STARTING POSITION: Assume a regular stance that's comfortably wide with a kettlebell placed between your feet. You may angle your toes slightly outward if this is more comfortable for your knees.

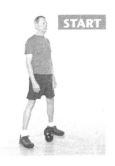
START

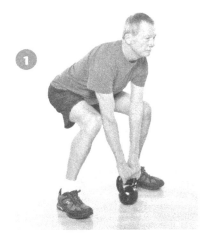

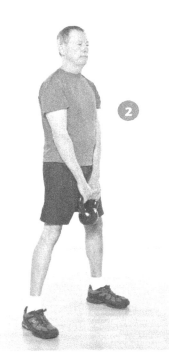

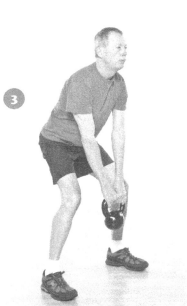

1 Keeping your back straight and your head high, squat down and grab the handle with a side-to-side grip.

2 Squeezing your butt and thigh muscles, stand up tall.

3 Lower into a squat. Use the power of your thighs, not your back.

STARTING POSITION: Assume a regular stance that's comfortably wide with the kettlebell placed just outside your right foot. You may angle your toes slightly outward if this is more comfortable for your knees.

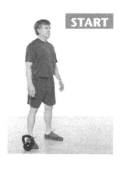

START

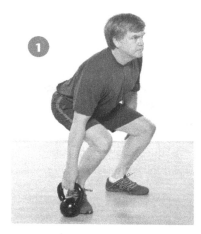

1 Lower your rear end into a squat until your thighs are parallel with the floor, and grab the bell using a right overhand grip.

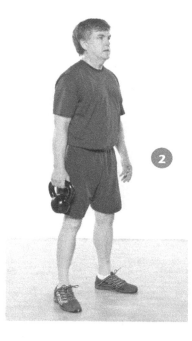

2 Stand up, keeping your arm at your side. Do not hold your breath.

3 Lower into a squat. Use the power of your thighs, not your back.

Repeat, then switch sides.

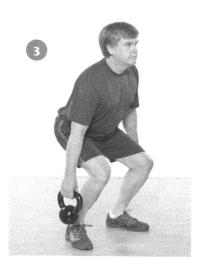

STARTING POSITION: Assume a regular stance that's comfortably wide with a kettlebell placed just outside each foot. You may angle your toes slightly outward if this is more comfortable for your knees.

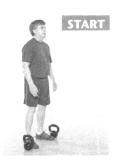

START

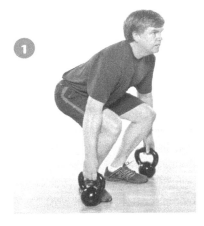

1

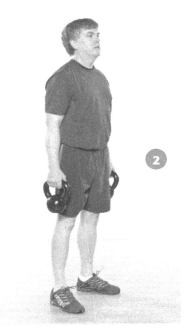

2

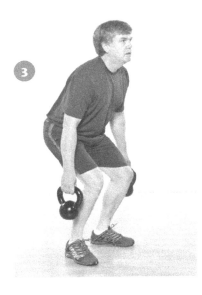

3

1 Lower your rear end into a squat until your thighs are parallel with the floor, and grab a bell in each hand using an overhand grip.

2 Stand up, keeping your arms by your sides.

3 Take a deep breath and exhale as you lower into a squat. Use the power of your thighs, not your back.

Return to upright position.

single-bell racked squat

Before you can do a racked squat, you need to know how to rack your bell (see page 23).

STARTING POSITION: Assume a regular stance that's comfortably wide with the kettlebell placed just outside your right foot. You may angle your toes slightly outward if this is more comfortable for your knees.

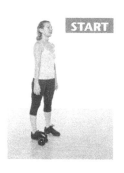

START

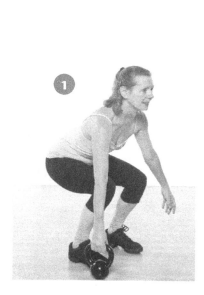

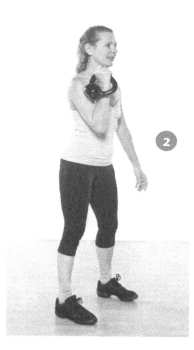

1–2 Lower your rear end into a squat until your thighs are parallel with the floor, and grab the bell in your right hand. Stand up, keeping your arm at your side, and move the bell to rack position at your right shoulder. Protect your wrist by maintaining neutral wrist position; your grip should be relaxed.

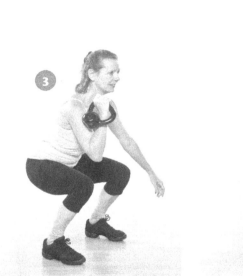

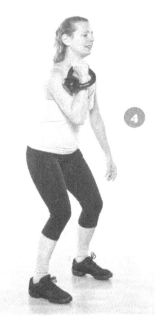

3 Lower into a squat.

4 Use the power of your legs to stand up.

Repeat, then switch sides.

VARIATION: This can also be done with two bells.

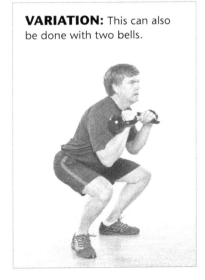

You can start with a heavier bell with this squat.

STARTING POSITION: Stand with your feet together and hold a kettlebell in both hands using a side-by-side grip.

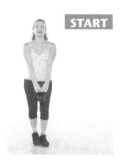

START

1–2 Step sideways to the left with your left foot, keep everything facing forward, and squat down, getting your thighs parallel and touching the kettlebell to the floor if possible.

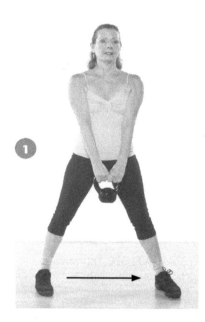

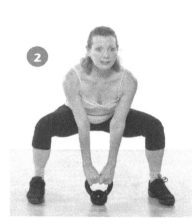

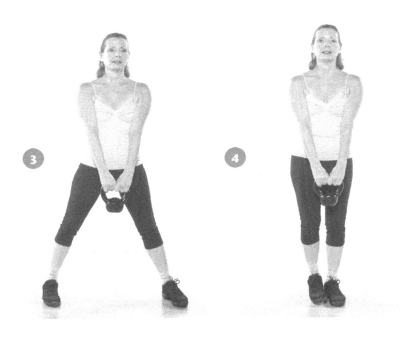

3 Use the power of your legs to stand up.

4 Step your left foot back to starting position.

Step to the right with your right foot and perform a squat.

Continue alternating sides.

deadlift series

Avoid this series if you have low back issues. To make sure you can do this safely, practice this move without a kettlebell first, or place the kettlebell on a table or block so you don't have to extend back so much. Don't bounce or overstretch, and don't jerk the bell off the floor.

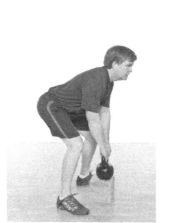 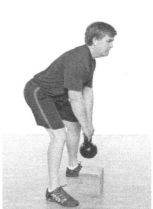 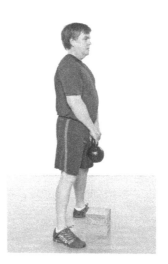

Block modification

Traditionally this move is performed with heavy weights. I don't recommend that until you know how your body responds. Instead, perform this slowly a few times without a kettlebell until you know your body can handle the move. The deadlift is done from the hip hinge joint, not by the rounding of the back.

Caution: This is a controversial move so if you decide to perform it, be careful and do so slowly.

STARTING POSITION: Assume a regular stance with your feet a little wider apart than normal.

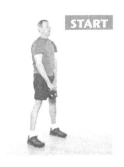

START

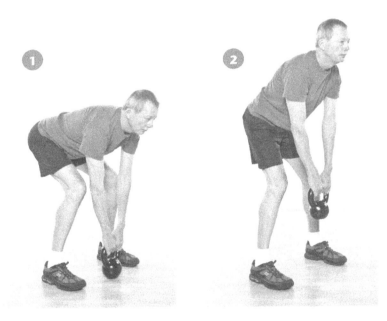

1 Keeping your back straight from the base of your skull to the base of your tailbone (a yardstick should be able to rest flat on your back), bend at the hip hinge joint, only going as far as your hamstrings will allow. Don't bounce or overstretch.

2 Engage your gluteal muscles—not your back—to slowly return to standing.

Start with a lighter kettlebell, watch your form in a mirror and avoid rounding your back.

STARTING POSITION: Stand with your feet together and place the kettlebell just outside your right foot.

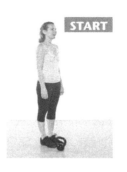

START

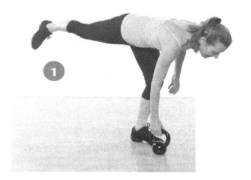

1 Bending over from the hip hinge joint, grab the handle using a right thumb-up or overhand grip. Extend your right leg straight back to counterbalance. Keep your hips level to the floor.

2–3 Engaging your torso and gluteal muscles, slowly return to starting position.

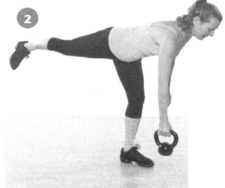

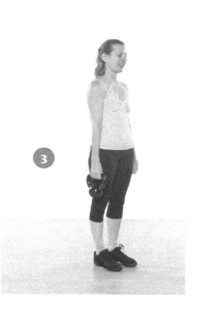

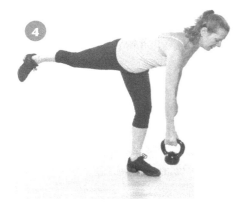

4 Bend over from the hip hinge joint again to return the bell to the floor.

Repeat, then switch sides.

MODIFICATION: To reduce the distance, raise the bell's height by placing it on blocks or a stack of thick books.

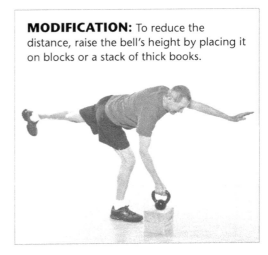

STARTING POSITION: Assume a regular stance and hold a kettlebell in each hand, arms along your sides.

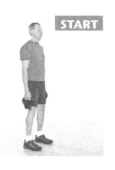

START

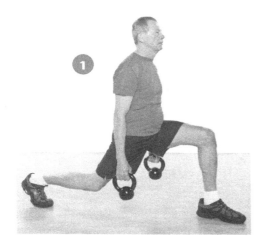

1 Lunge a comfortable distance forward with your left leg. Bend your right knee toward the floor, allowing your heel to come off the floor. Keep your front knee pointed in the same direction as your foot, but don't let it extend over your toes. Pay attention to your low back posture.

2 Return to starting position.

Perform with your other leg and continue alternating legs.

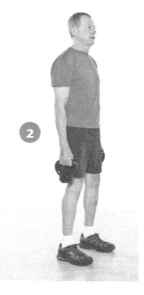

VARIATION: This can also be done by stepping backward into a lunge.

STARTING POSITION: Assume a staggered stance with a bell held in rack position at each shoulder. Allow your rear heel to lift off the ground.

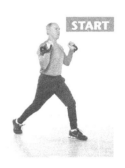

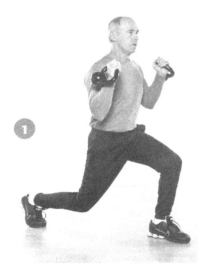

1 Slowly bend both knees, bringing your rear knee toward the floor. Keep your front knee pointed in the same direction as your foot, but don't let it extend over your toes. Pay attention to your low back posture.

2 Return to starting position.

Repeat, then switch sides.

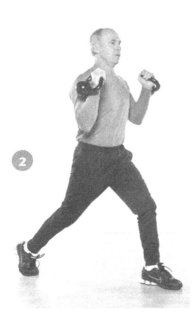

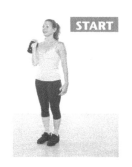

START

Caution: If you have high blood pressure or heart issues, holding a kettlebell overhead might be ill-advised.

STARTING POSITION: Assume a regular stance and hold the kettlebell with your right hand in rack position.

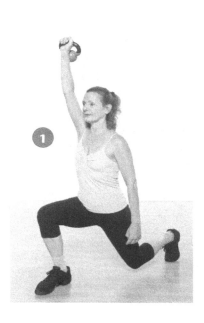

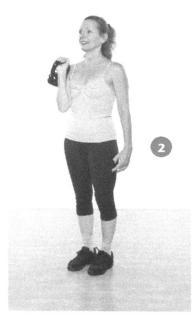

1 Press the bell overhead to lockout position, keeping your wrist in proper position, and lunge a comfortable distance forward with your left leg. Keep your knees, hips and torso pointed in the same direction as your feet throughout the movement. Bend your right knee toward the floor, allowing your heel to come off the floor.

2 Return to starting position.

Repeat, then switch sides.

VARIATION: This can also be done by stepping backward into a lunge.

ADVANCED: Hold a kettlebell in each hand and alternate the overhead press with each lunge.

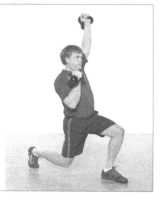

Because you'll be generating extra power with your legs, you can use a heavier bell if your joints can tolerate it. Remember to breathe properly with each rep, exhaling when pressing upward.

STARTING POSITION: Assume a regular stance and hold the kettlebell with your right hand in rack position.

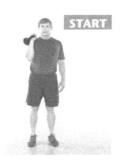

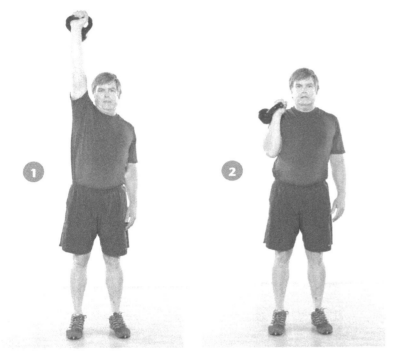

1 Slightly bend your knees then use your legs to transfer the power up through your hips and pelvis and into your shoulder and arm to press the bell up while turning your palm forward. Hold for a moment, keeping your arm above your hips and elbow straight.

2 Return to starting position.

Repeat, then switch sides.

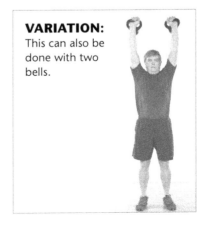

VARIATION: This can also be done with two bells.

Because you'll be generating extra power with your legs, you can use heavier bells if your joints can tolerate it. Remember to breathe properly with each rep, exhaling when pressing upward.

STARTING POSITION: Assume a regular stance with a slight bend in your knees and hold a bell in rack position in each hand.

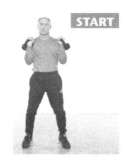

START

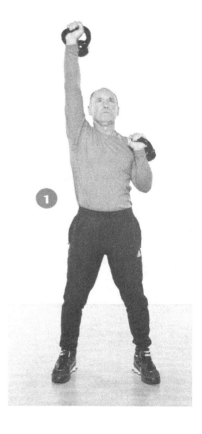

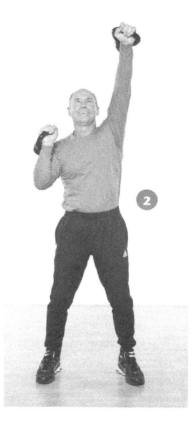

1 Press the right bell overhead while turning your palm forward (you may bend your knees slightly to assist in powering up the bell). Hold for a moment.

2 Return to starting position then press the left bell overhead while turning your palm forward. Hold for a moment.

Continue alternating arms.

STARTING POSITION: Assume a wide stance and hold a kettlebell in both hands using a side-by-side grip. Keep your arms extended in front of your hips.

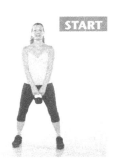

START

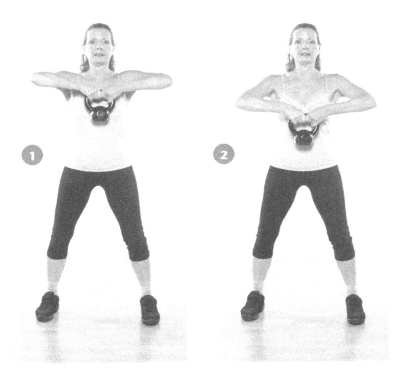

1 Keeping the bell close to your body, pull it up to chest height. Your elbows will come out to the sides.

2 Lower the bell to starting position.

STARTING POSITION: Assume a regular stance and hold a bell in each hand, arms by your sides.

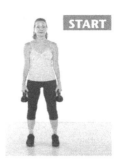

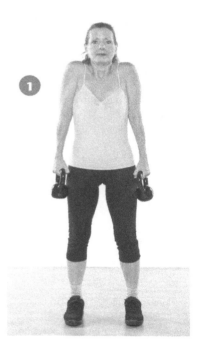

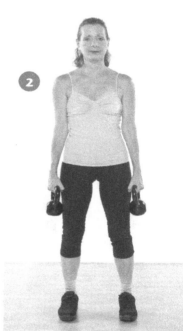

1 Shrug your shoulders up to your ears and hold for a moment.

2 Release to starting position.

STARTING POSITION: Assume a staggered stance with your right leg forward. Bending at the waist about 45 degrees, place your right hand on your right thigh for support and grasp the handle with your left hand. Keeping your arm extended, bring the bell off the ground.

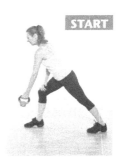
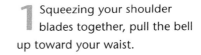

1 Squeezing your shoulder blades together, pull the bell up toward your waist.

2 Extend your arm toward the floor.

Repeat, then switch sides.

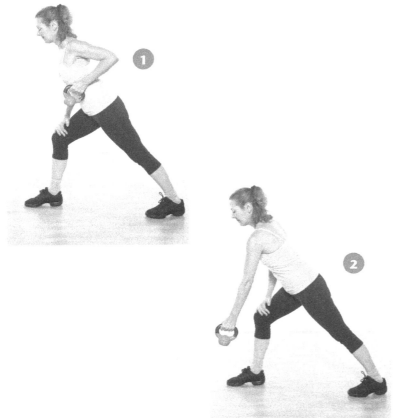

bent-over triceps extension

STARTING POSITION: Assume a staggered stance with your left leg forward. Bending at the waist about 45 degrees, place your left hand on your left thigh for support and grasp the handle with your right hand, thumb up. Squeezing your shoulder blades together, pull the bell up toward your chest until your arm makes a 90-degree angle and your elbow is next to your ribs.

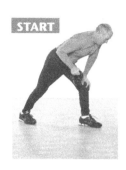

START

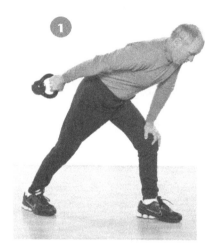

1

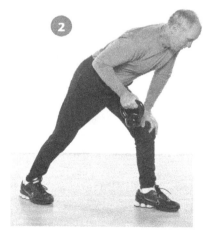

2

1 Keeping your right elbow next to your ribs, extend your arm straight back.

2 Return to starting position.

Repeat, then switch sides.

Use this movement to learn how to control and stop a moving weight.

STARTING POSITION: Assume a regular stance and hold the kettlebell with a right overhand grip, positioning the bell at your left hip.

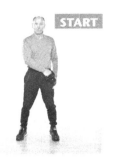

START

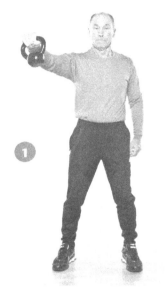

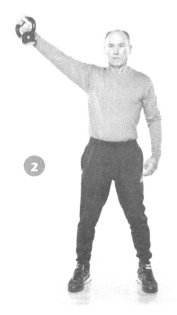

1–2 Keeping your arm straight but not locked, swing the bell diagonally up and across your body to full extension. Hold momentarily.

3 Return to starting position.

Repeat, then switch arms.

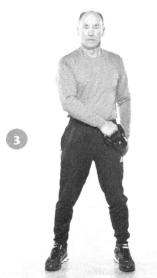

VARIATION: You can also perform this by rotating your torso, moving your hips and shoulders as a unit with a pivoting motion of your feet.

STARTING POSITION: Assume a plank (high push-up) position with your hands beneath your shoulders and your legs extended straight back behind you. Position the kettlebell under your sternum.

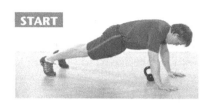
START

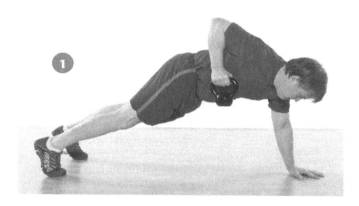
1

1 Balancing on your left hand and keeping your body as parallel to the floor as possible, grab the bell with your right hand and pull it to your waist. Focus on not rotating your torso by engaging your abs and glutes.

2 Return the bell to the floor.

Repeat, then switch sides.

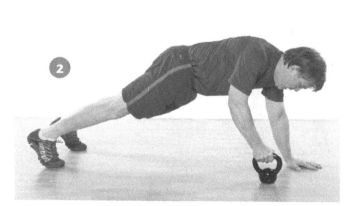
2

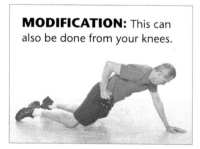

MODIFICATION: This can also be done from your knees.

This advanced exercise challenges the total kinetic chain and, when done correctly, recruits total-body engagement from the calf muscles to the neck in addition to the core.

STARTING POSITION: Assume a plank (high push-up) position with your hands beneath your shoulders and your legs extended straight back behind you. Place the kettlebell under your sternum.

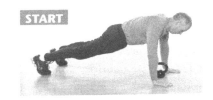

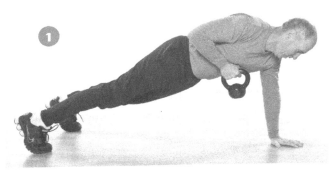

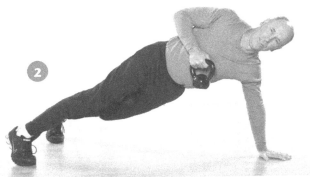

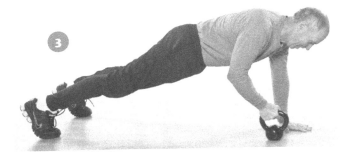

1 Balancing on your left hand and keeping your body as parallel to the floor as possible, grab the bell with your right hand and pull it to your chest.

2 Rotate your body to the right, keeping the bell in front of your sternum, until your shoulders are stacked.

3 Return the bell to the floor.

Now grab the bell with your left hand and perform the same move in the opposite direction. Continue alternating between left and right hands.

plank rotation with arm extension
target: full body

This advanced exercise challenges the total kinetic chain and, when done correctly, recruits total-body engagement from the calf muscles to the neck, with special emphasis on the arm and shoulders as well as the core and upper back muscles, which are used as stabilizers. Practice this move without a bell first or a very light kettlebell. Form is critical!

Caution: Avoid this exercise if you have back or shoulder concerns.

STARTING POSITION: Assume a plank (high push-up) position with your hands beneath your shoulders and your legs extended straight back behind you. Place the kettlebell under your sternum.

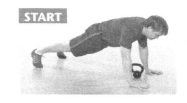

START

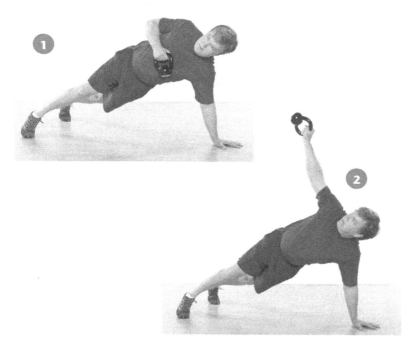

1–2 Grab the bell with your right hand and rotate your body to the right as the bell moves up and over your right shoulder. Your body should nearly be at right angles to the floor.

3 Return the bell to the floor and switch sides.

Continue alternating between left and right hands.

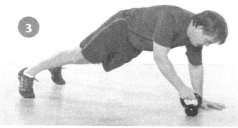

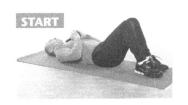

You may want to do this on an exercise mat to provide some cushioning for your back.

Caution: Avoid this exercise if you have back or neck issues.

STARTING POSITION: Lie on your back with your knees bent and feet flat on the floor. Grasp the ball of the bell firmly with both hands and rest it on your chest.

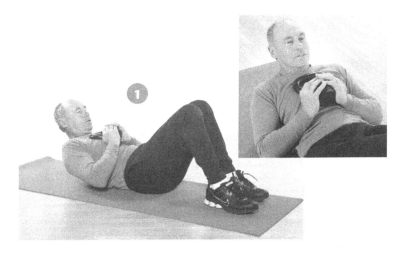

1 Tuck your chin toward your chest as you curl your shoulders off the floor.

2 Slowly return to starting position.

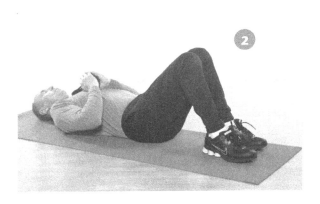

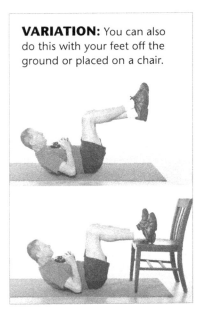

VARIATION: You can also do this with your feet off the ground or placed on a chair.

floor series

target: thighs, glutes

If you have sensitive knees, place a mat under your kneeling knee.

STARTING POSITION: Kneel on your right knee and place your left foot in front of you on the floor. Hold a bell in rack position in front of each shoulder.

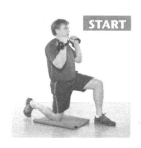
START

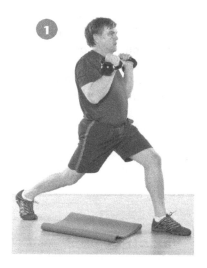
1

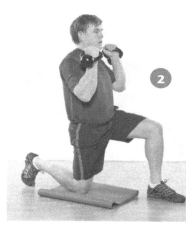
2

1 Stand up, staying mindful of the mechanics of your low back and knees.

2 Return to kneeling position.

Repeat, then switch sides.

MODIFICATION: You can also try this with a light kettlebell or no weight at all.

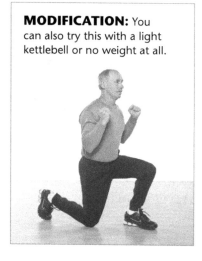

If you have sensitive knees, place a mat under your kneeling knee. Do not do this advanced move until you can do the Double-Bell Kneeling Get-Up (page 74).

STARTING POSITION: Kneel on your right knee and place your left foot in front of you on the floor. Hold the bell in rack position in front of your left shoulder.

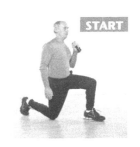

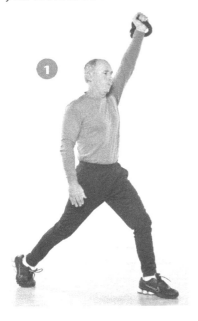

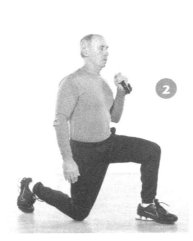

1 Stand up and press the bell overhead, rotating your hand forward.

2 Return to kneeling position.

Repeat, then switch sides.

DOUBLE-BELL VARIATION: This can also be performed with two bells held in rack position.

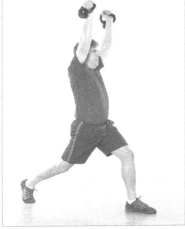

This is an advanced exercise. You may want to do this on an exercise mat to provide some cushioning for your back and tailbone.

Caution: Avoid this exercise if you have back or neck issues.

STARTING POSITION: Sit on the floor with your knees bent and feet flat on the floor. Hold the handle of the bell with both hands at your chest.

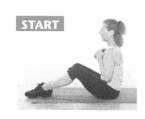

START

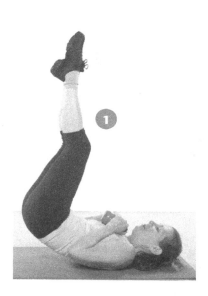

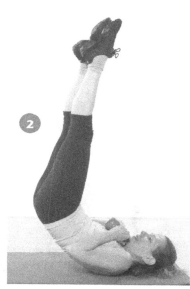

1 Keeping the bell next to your chest and engaging your core, roll back, allowing your hips to lift off the floor.

2 As your hips come off the floor, extend your feet toward the ceiling, pointing your toes and keeping your legs as straight as possible.

Roll back to starting position.

ROCKING HORSE WITH PRESS: For an advanced challenge, press the bell toward the ceiling as you roll back, keeping the bell over your chest.

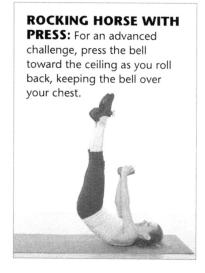

compound series

The exercises in this series are more complex and are often called "compound exercises" because they include multiple movements and target several muscles. Make sure you can perform the individual components with correct form before combining the movements and/or introducing heavier bells.

arm curl & leg curl
target: biceps, hamstrings, core

STARTING POSITION: Stand with your feet together and hold a bell in each hand in front of your body with an overhand grip, arms straight yet relaxed. Your palms should face forward.

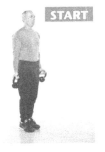

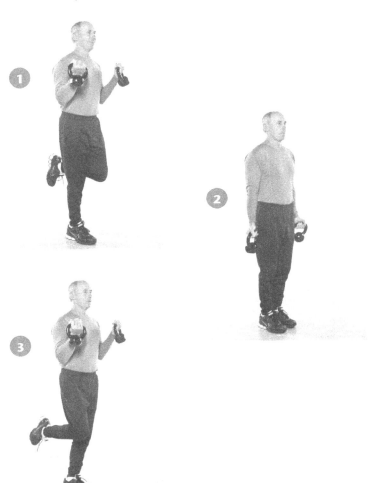

1 Inhale and curl the bell to rack position as you simultaneously curl your left leg toward your left buttock.

2 Exhale and return to starting position.

3 Perform the arm curl, this time curling the opposite leg.

SINGLE-BELL VARIATION: This can also be performed with one bell. Remember to switch the bell to the other hand at some point.

alternating single-arm pull

target: shoulders, trapezius, biceps

STARTING POSITION: Assume an athletic short-stop position and hold the kettlebell with an overhand grip.

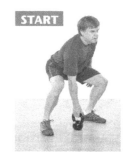
START

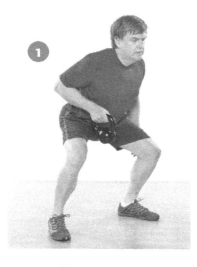
1

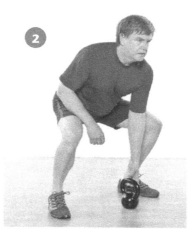
2

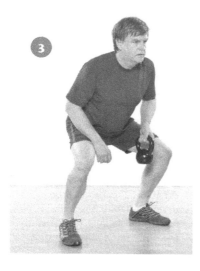
3

1 Pull the bell up toward your chest.

2 Lower your arm and switch hands at the bottom.

3 Pull the bell up toward your chest.

Continue alternating arms.

Since this is primarily a shoulder/arm exercise, use a lighter bell.

STARTING POSITION: Assume a regular stance with a slightly wider stance if need be, and hold a kettlebell in each hand using an overhand grip, keeping your arms alongside your body.

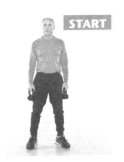

START

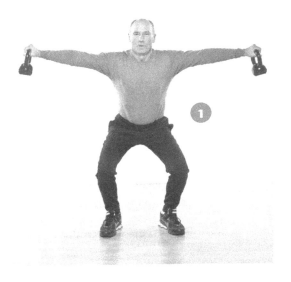

1 Perform a half squat and lift the bells out to the sides, no higher than shoulder level. Hold momentarily.

2 Return to starting position.

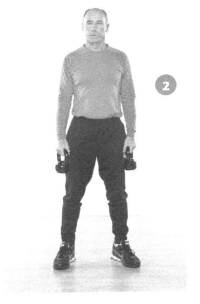

VARIATION: You can also hold the kettlebell in one hand and pass the bell from hand to hand as you stand up.

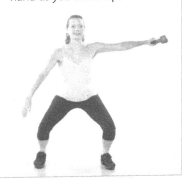

STARTING POSITION: Assume a regular stance and hold the bell in rack position at your right shoulder.

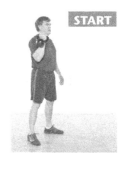

START

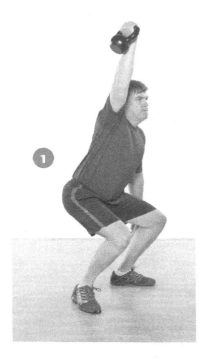

1

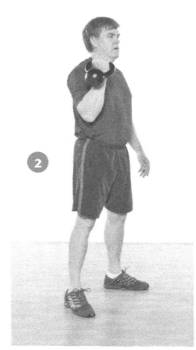

2

1 Inhale as you squat down halfway and press the bell directly overhead, turning your palm forward as you press. Hold momentarily.

2 Exhale as you return to starting position.

Repeat, then switch sides.

VARIATION: This can also be done with two bells.

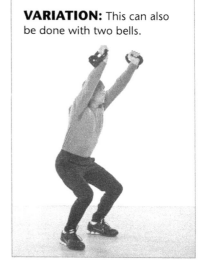

STARTING POSITION: Assume a regular stance and grab a kettlebell in each hand using an overhand grip, keeping your arms at your sides, palms facing in.

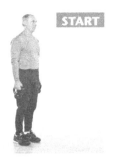

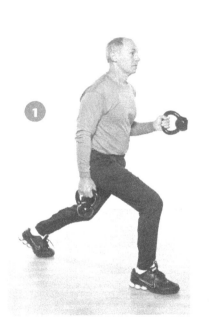

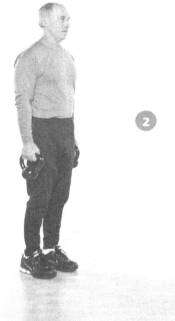

1 Lunge forward with your right leg, bending your rear knee to the floor, if possible. At the same time, bend your left elbow 90 degrees—you'll look like an old-time gunslinger.

2 Return to starting position. Repeat, rest and then switch leg position.

VARIATION: You can also lunge backward.

DOUBLE-BELL VARIATION: This can also be done with two bells.

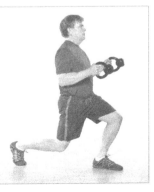

swing series

Swing movements are unique to kettlebell training in that they engage the total-body kinetic chain. Most conventional weight-training exercises focus on controlled concentric and eccentric contractions while working through the full range of motion. A kettlebell workout is much like performing Olympic lifts—dynamic and explosive. Swings are where the momentum concept comes into play. When you do a swing, you'll engage your legs, butt and hips, as well as your torso; your arms really only serve as a fulcrum. The beauty of swing moves is that they engage prime mover muscles as well as deep-lying stabilizers. The advantage of kettlebell swings for 50+ folks is that very often as we get older, not only do we lose muscle mass and strength, we lose what's called fast-twitch muscle fibers even more. Swings, when performed safely, foster development of fast-twitch muscle fiber development, which will slow down the decline of your reaction time.

Keep in mind that a body in motion tends to stay in motion, and if you can't maintain control of the kinetic chain, pain will invade your body. Often the reason people get hurt while performing kettlebell swings is because the weaker deep-lying muscles have never been trained prior to a kettlebell workout.

Swings will help you improve power but learning and practicing the correct technique is critical. It's also important to learn how to slow down a kettlebell too, otherwise you'll be thrown off balance or your joints will be taken past a safe range of motion, injuring the supporting joints and muscles. If you don't believe this, imagine trying to catch yourself while falling.

Swings are very advanced moves. I strongly believe you need to have a solid foundation of muscular endurance, strength and coordination before you should engage in them since they allow you to lift more weight than you could without momentum. Don't overdo it! Ironically, in traditional weight training, a good trainer never allows you to swing the weights (this is called cheating), but using momentum in certain kettlebell movements is okay. Start slowly and with a light weight.

Make sure you have a firm grip on the bell and that the area around you is free of things and people. You may use gloves or chalk to secure the kettlebell.

STARTING POSITION: Assume a regular stance. Place the kettlebell with its handle angled 45 degrees between your legs.

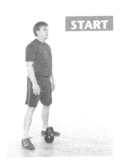

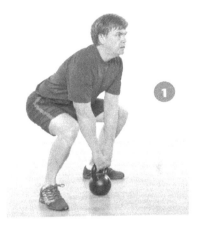

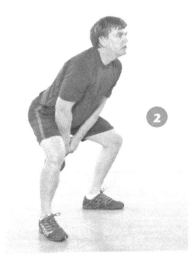

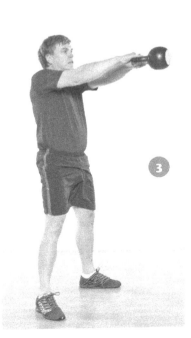

1 Lower your hips back and down to squat and grasp the handle with both hands using an overhand grip. Your arms and torso should move as a unit.

2–3 Hike the bell back between your legs and then contract the muscles of your hips and legs simultaneously while you stand up straight and allow the bell to swing forward to chest or head height. Keep your arms extended.

continued on next page

continued from previous page

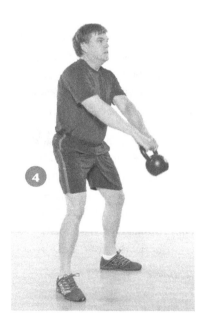

4 Allow gravity to bring the bell back between your legs but control its downward motion.

Quickly reverse the direction upward again.

You may use gloves or chalk to secure the kettlebell. Some people like to place the free arm out to the side, on the hip or behind the back; experiment to see which provides the most control and counterbalance for you.

STARTING POSITION: Place the kettlebell with its handle angled 45 degrees between your legs.

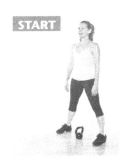

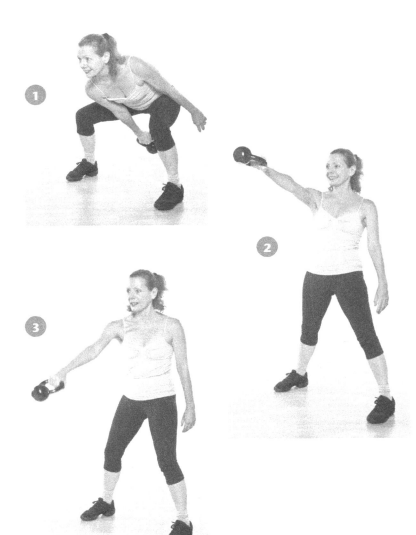

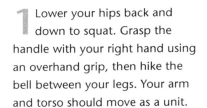

1 Lower your hips back and down to squat. Grasp the handle with your right hand using an overhand grip, then hike the bell between your legs. Your arm and torso should move as a unit.

2 Contract the muscles of your hips and legs simultaneously while you stand up straight and allow the bell to swing forward to chest or head height. Keep your arm extended.

3 Allow gravity to bring the bell back between your legs but control its downward motion.

Quickly reverse the direction upward again. Repeat, then switch arms.

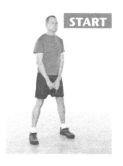

STARTING POSITION: Assume an athletic stance and hold the kettlebell in both hands using a side-by-side grip.

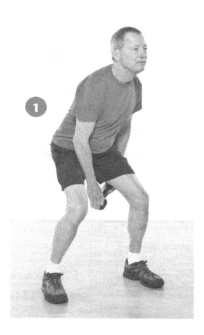

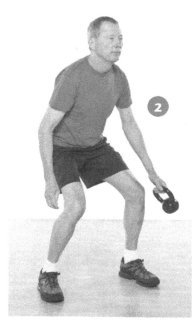

1–4 Squat slightly to pass the kettlebell under, around and through your legs several times. Make the transition slowly at first and progress to a quicker transfer from hand to hand. Be careful not to drop the bell!

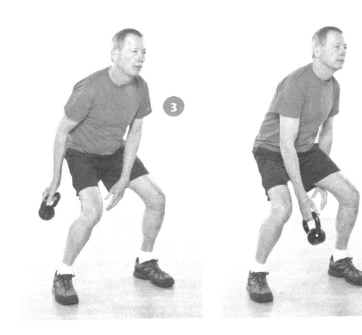

Once you've done this several times, reverse direction. When you're done, stand up straight to stretch your back muscles (the Double Wood Chop stretch, page 107, works well).

alternating swing & catch

This very challenging advanced kettlebell exercise emphasizes hand-eye coordination. Make sure you've mastered the basic swings before trying this—swings should be done without any shoulder or low back discomfort. Start with a light bell—this exercise can be dangerous if you drop the bell. In addition, you must control the motion at all times—don't let the bell take you into un-safe zones. This exercise demands good grip strength; gloves are highly recommended.

STARTING POSITION: Straddle the bell with your feet slightly wider than your shoulders, squat slightly and grasp the handle with a right overhand grip. Keep your arm straight but not locked throughout the movement.

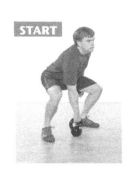

START

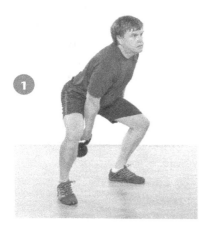

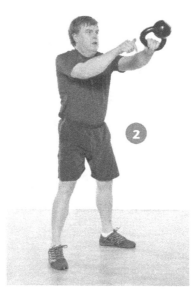

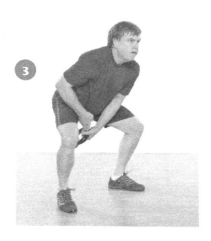

1 Gently swing the bell several times to prepare the body and generate some momentum.

2 As the bell reaches its apex (between shoulder and eye height), quickly release the bell and re-grab the handle with your left hand. The height at which you release the bell is based upon your vision and reaction time.

3 As the kettlebell comes back down, decelerate the motion by squatting down and bending slightly at your hips and knees, allowing the bell to go between your legs.

Continue swinging the bell back up while coming to an upright posture, engaging your core and leg muscles and switching hands at the apex of each upward swing.

clean series

Often as a person get older, explosive power declines. If you're healthy, this series is an excellent way to maintain your explosive power; in some cases it'll improve. The clean is an advanced movement that takes the kettlebell off the floor and to the shoulder using a light upward swing. Learn the motion with a light weight first. You may want to only do one rep at a time and rest and re-group between reps. Some people complain that the kettlebell hitting the forearm bothers them. If you're banging the bell on your forearms, you're probably swinging the bell too far. Pay attention to your form and body mechanics. If this continues to bother you, avoid this exercise or wear something to protect your forearms.

basic clean   target: *full body, fast-twitch muscles*

STARTING POSITION: Assume a regular or wide stance with the kettlebell slightly out in front of your body and between your legs, handle angled 45 degrees.

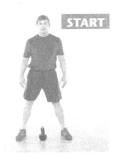

START

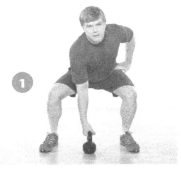

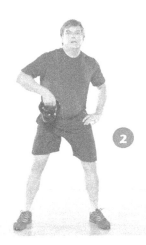

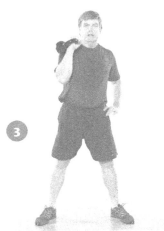

1 Lower your hips backward and down and grasp the handle with an overhand grip.

2–3 Perform a light upward swing, moving the arm and torso as a single unit; when the bell reaches waist height, bend your elbow to bring your hand to your shoulder and loosen your grip to allow the bell to flip over. The bell should end up in rack position.

Push the bell off your forearm, flip the handle and return to starting position.

The goal of this exercise is to teach the body to work as a team by recruiting your whole body in a systematic fashion to generate power.

STARTING POSITION: Assume a regular or wide stance with the kettlebell slightly out in front of your body and between your legs, handle angled 45 degrees.

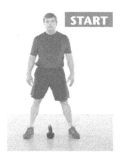

START

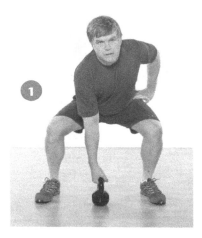

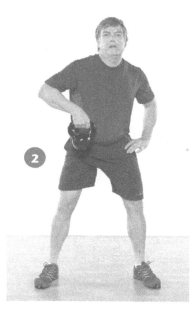

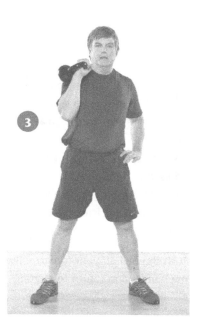

1 Lower your hips backward and down and grasp the handle with an overhand grip.

2–3 Perform a light upward swing, moving the arm and torso as a single unit; when the bell reaches waist height, bend your elbow to bring your hand to your shoulder and loosen your grip to allow the bell to flip over. The bell should end up in rack position for a short moment.

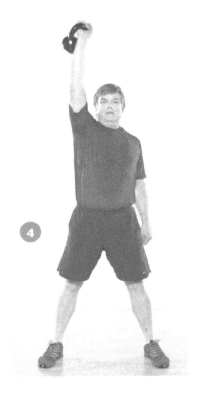

4 Bend your knees to "drop" under the bell and then drive up through your feet, extending your legs and pressing the kettlebell upward.

Return to starting position with control.

ADVANCED: When you're comfortable with this movement, you can step backward/forward as you press the bell upward.

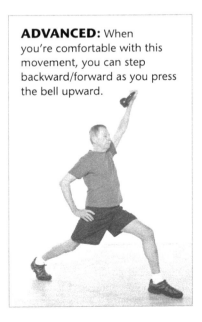

STARTING POSITION: Stand with your legs together and arms by your sides.

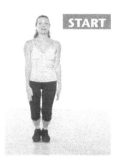

START

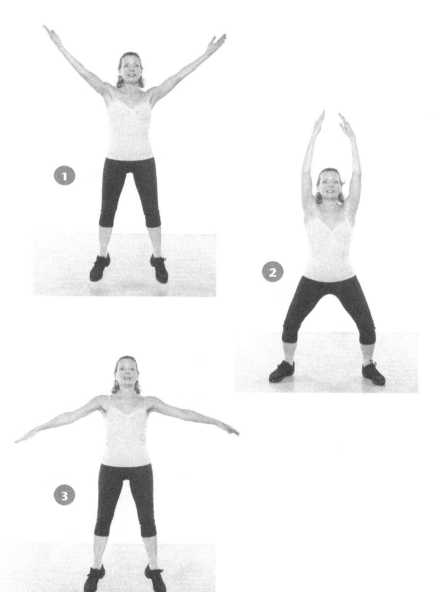

1–3 Without stopping, jump your feet apart as you raise your arms to the ceiling, then jump your feet back to starting position and bring your arms to your sides.

Continue jumping.

STARTING POSITION: Stand tall with good posture.

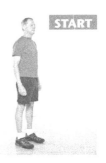

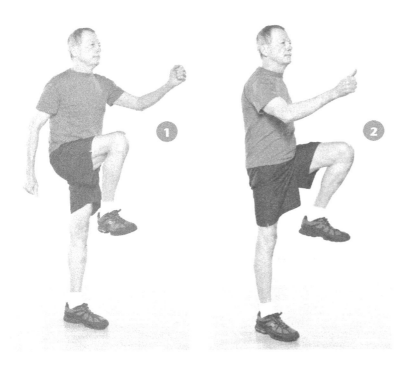

1–2 March in place, gradually lifting your knees higher as you warm up. As you limber up, swing your arms in opposition as you lift your knees.

Continue for 1–3 minutes or longer.

STARTING POSITION: Assume a regular stance that's comfortably wide. You may angle your toes slightly outward if this is more comfortable for your knees.

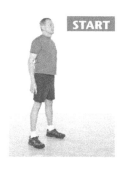

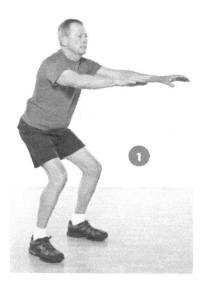

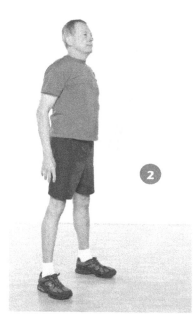

1 Keeping your back straight and your head high, lower into a partial squat. You can raise your arms for balance if necessary.

2 Squeezing your butt and thigh muscles, stand up tall.

3 Once you're ready, you can squat lower, until your thighs are parallel to the floor. Use the power of your thighs, not your back, and don't let your knees extend past your toes.

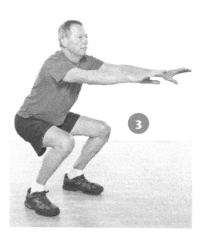

STARTING POSITION: Assume a regular stance with your hands on your hips.

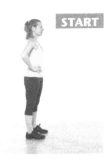

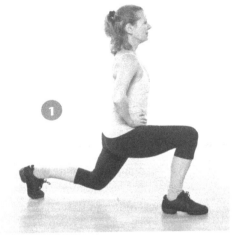

1 Lunge a comfortable distance forward with your right leg. Bend your left knee toward the floor, allowing your heel to come off the floor. Keep your front knee pointed in the same direction as your foot, but don't let it extend over your toes. Pay attention to your low back posture.

2 Return to starting position.

Perform with your other leg and continue alternating legs.

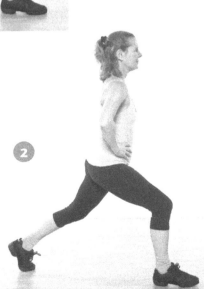

VARIATION: This can also be done by stepping backward into a lunge.

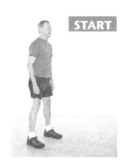

START

The deadlift is done from the hip hinge joint, not by the rounding of the back.

Caution: This is a controversial move so if you decide to perform it, be careful and do so slowly.

STARTING POSITION: Assume a regular stance with your feet a little wider apart than normal.

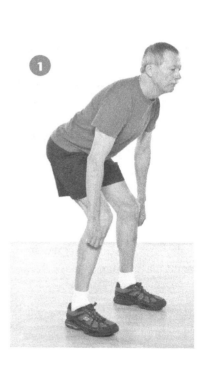

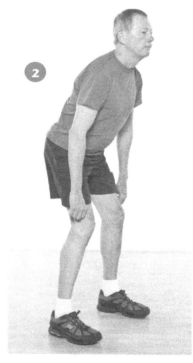

1 Keeping your back straight from the base of your skull to the base of your tailbone (a yardstick should be able to rest flat on your back), bend at the hip hinge joint, only going as far as your hamstrings will allow. Don't bounce or overstretch.

2 Engage your gluteal muscles—not your back—to slowly return to standing.

Caution: Perform this move slowly and with control. If you have neck issues, get clearance from your doctor before doing this.

STARTING POSITION: Stand tall with your arms along your sides.

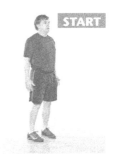

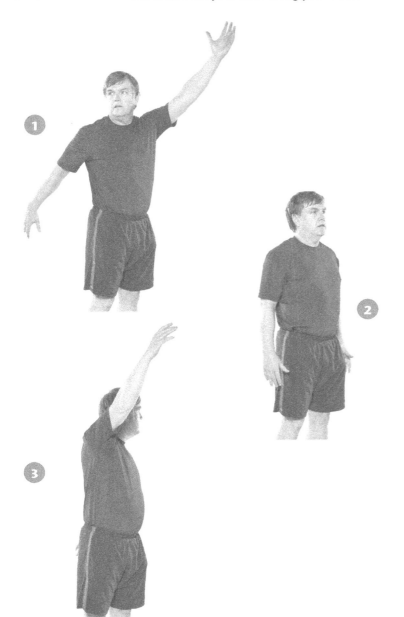

1 Gently swing your left arm forward as you swing your right arm backward, moving your arms as high as they can easily go. Gently look to the right.

2 Return to starting position.

3 Gently swing your right arm forward and look to the left while your right arm moves backward.

STARTING POSITION: Assume a regular stance and raise both arms out to the sides at shoulder height.

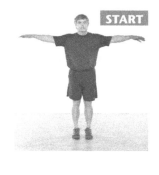

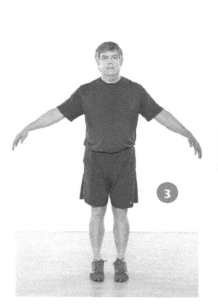

1–3 Keeping your arms straight, slowly circle your arms forward, starting with small circles and progressing to larger ones.

Reverse direction.

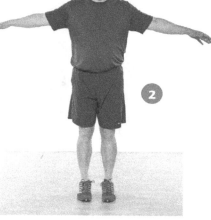

THE POSITION: From kneeling, place your forearms on the mat so that your elbows are beneath your shoulders and your forearms point forward. When you're ready, extend your legs back, resting your weight in the balls of your feet and your forearms. Your body should form a straight line from head to heels. Hold as tolerated. Do not hold your breath; do not raise your rear end.

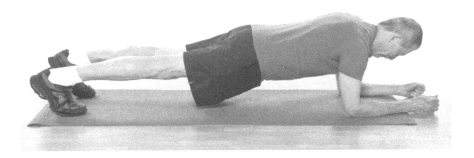

MODIFICATION: This can also be performed from your knees.

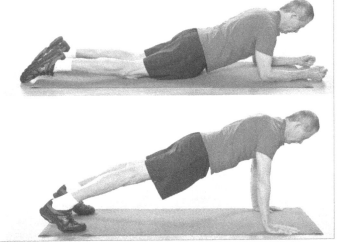

VARIATION: This can also be performed from a high push-up position, with your hands on the floor beneath your shoulders.

This is an advanced move in which proper alignment is critical.

Caution: Avoid this move if you have shoulder issues.

THE POSITION: Lie on your left side with your left elbow under your left shoulder. Stack your right shoulder over your left shoulder, right hip over left hip, right knee over left knee and right ankle over left ankle. When you're ready, lift your hips off the ground, forming a straight line from your head to your ankles. Hold as tolerated. Do not hold your breath.

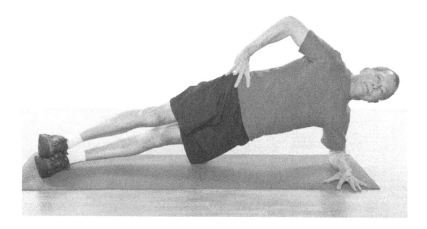

MODIFICATION: Bend the top knee and step it in front or behind you to reduce the challenge.

Caution: If you have a history of neck problems (e.g., herniated discs, arthritis of the neck), consult a health professional before performing this move.

STARTING POSITION: Stand with proper posture.

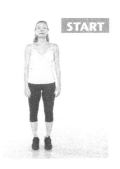

1 While inhaling deeply through your nose, slowly tilt your head to the left. Once in this position, place the fingertips of your left hand on the right side of your head. While exhaling through your lips, gently pull your head to your left shoulder. Keep your shoulders relaxed and down. Hold this position and continue to breathe deeply in through your nose and out through your lips.

2 Release and return to starting position before switching sides.

3 Inhale slowly through your nose and look to your left as far as you can without feeling discomfort. Exhale slowly through your lips and hold this position for a moment, feeling the stretch.

4 Inhale slowly through your nose and look slowly to the right. Exhale slowly through your lips and hold this position for a moment, feeling the stretch.

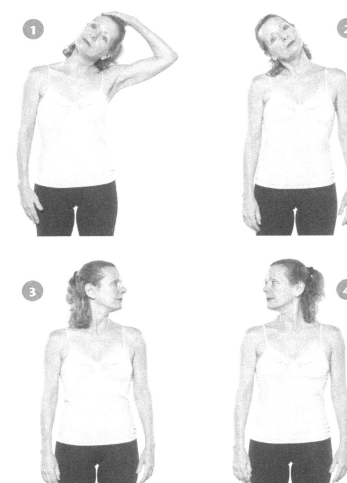

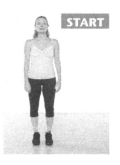

START

Caution: If you have a history of neck problems (e.g., herniated discs, arthritis of the neck), consult a health professional before performing this move.

STARTING POSITION: Stand with proper posture.

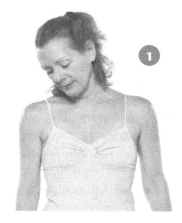

1

1–3 Slowly turn your head, tracing your chin along your collarbone. Perform several times in both directions.

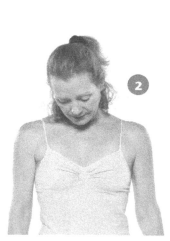

2

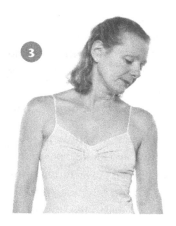

3

MODIFICATION: You can also try this stretch while sitting with proper posture in a stable chair.

Remember not to let your low back arch.

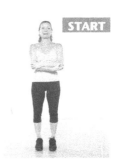

STARTING POSITION: Stand with proper posture. Place your right hand on your left elbow and your left hand on your right elbow.

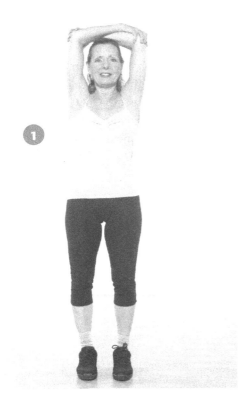

1 Slowly lift your arms overhead, raising them as high as feels comfortable. Hold the position for a moment. You are now framing your face in a picture frame created by your arms—smile.

MODIFICATION: You can also perform this while sitting in a stable chair.

stretches

STARTING POSITION: Stand with proper posture and place your hands behind your head.

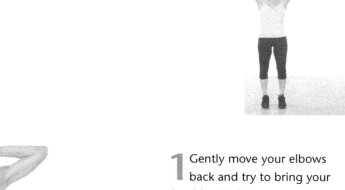

START

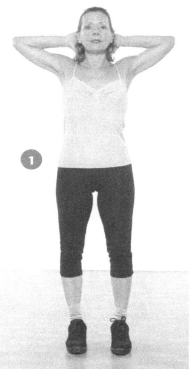

1 Gently move your elbows back and try to bring your shoulder blades together. Focus on opening up the chest and tightening the upper back muscles. Only go as far back as is comfortable and hold for a moment.

MODIFICATION: You can also perform this while sitting in a stable chair.

STARTING POSITION: Stand with proper posture and clasp your hands behind your back.

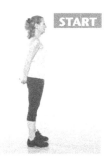

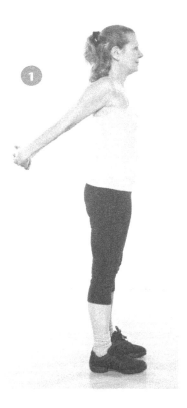

1 Raise both hands up behind you, feeling the stretch in your chest and the fronts of your shoulders. Only go up as high as is comfortable and hold for a moment.

stretches

elbow touch

target: shoulders, chest, upper back

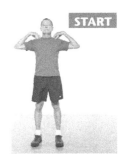

START

STARTING POSITION: Stand with proper posture and place your right hand on your right shoulder and your left hand on your left shoulder.

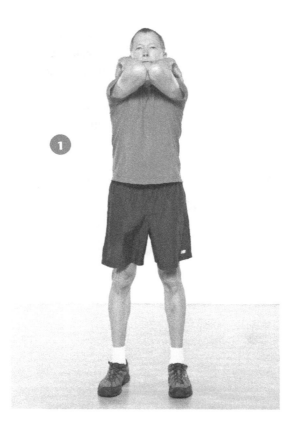

1 Gently move your elbows toward each other in front of your chest. Only move them as close as is comfortable and hold for a moment.

STARTING POSITION: Stand with proper posture. Position your hands in front of your body and interlace your fingers.

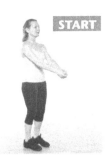

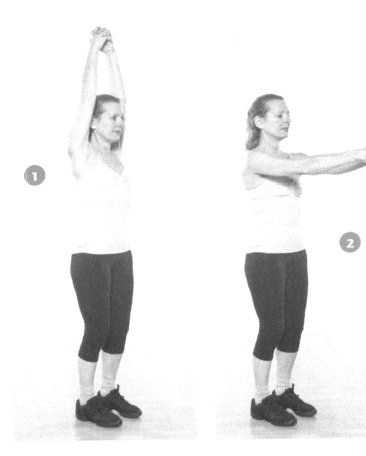

1 Inhale deeply through your nose and slowly raise both arms in front of you to a comfortable height. Hold 1–2 seconds.

2 Slowly lower your arms to starting position.

stretches
soup can pour
target: shoulders, rotator cuff

STARTING POSITION: Stand with proper posture, your arms at your sides and your palms facing back.

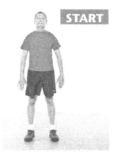

START

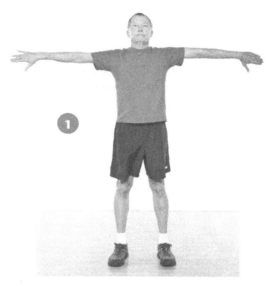

1 Inhale deeply through your nose and bring both arms slightly forward as you raise them out to the sides, keeping your palms facing back. Raise your arms no higher than shoulder level.

2 Exhale as you lower your arms.

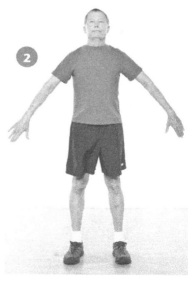

STARTING POSITION: Stand with proper posture with your arms at your sides. Squeeze a rolled-up towel or block between your right arm and your torso and bend your right elbow 90 degrees. Point your thumb up.

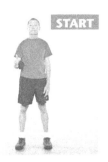

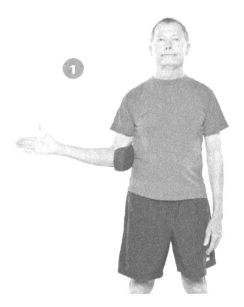

1 Keeping the towel against your body and your forearm parallel to the floor, rotate your forearm out to the side.

2 Rotate your forearm back in toward your body.

Repeat, then switch sides.

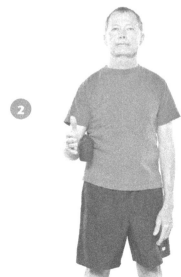

VARIATION: Try this with your palm facing down or up.

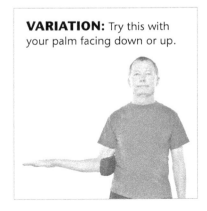

STARTING POSITION: Stand with proper posture. Raise your right hand to the ceiling and bring your left hand behind your back.

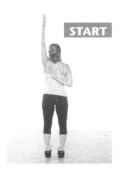

START

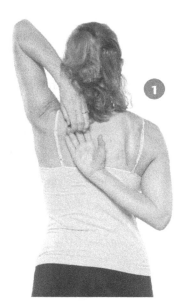

1 Bring your right hand down behind your head and clasp your fingers. Hold the position for a comfortable moment.

Release and switch sides.

MODIFICATION: If you have trouble grabbing your fingers, you can use a strap. Hold a strap in your right hand and raise your arm above your head; grab the other end with your other hand, palm facing out.

Raise your right hand up as high as possible to lift the lower hand, staying in your pain-free zone.

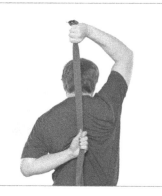

Caution: Avoid this exercise if you have poor balance. STOP if you notice undue compression in your knee or experience any low back discomfort. If you feel a cramp coming on, do a hamstrings stretch.

THE STRETCH: Stand with proper posture. Grab your right ankle with your right hand and bring your right heel toward your bottom. Keeping both knees as close together as possible, gently pull your heel closer to your bottom. Hold this stretch for a comfortable moment, then switch sides.

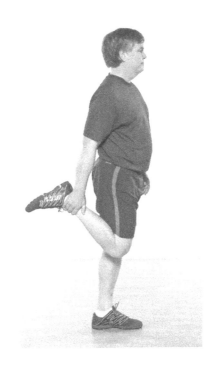

MODIFICATION: You can also stand by a chair, placing your hands on it for support. If you can't grab your foot with your hand, loop a strap around your ankle.

VARIATION: Raise your free arm toward the ceiling.

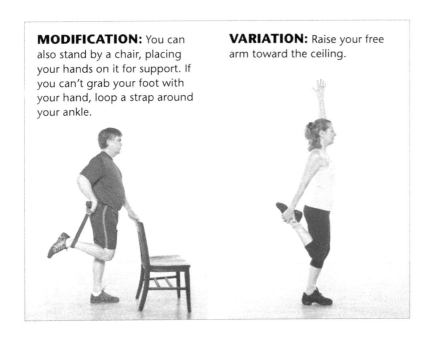

THE STRETCH: Stand tall. Keeping the heel down, slide your right leg as far back as you can. Bend your left knee until the desired stretch is felt in the calf area. Hold this stretch for a comfortable moment, then switch sides.

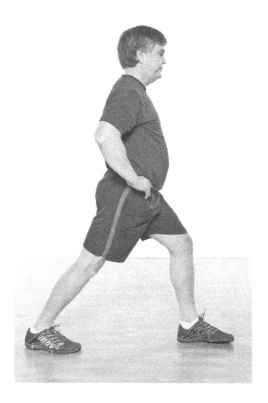

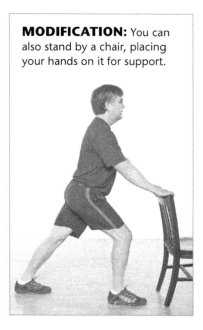

MODIFICATION: You can also stand by a chair, placing your hands on it for support.

STARTING POSITION: Rest on your hands and knees, keeping your hands under your shoulders and your knees under your hips. Keep your head neutral.

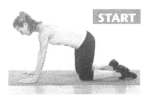

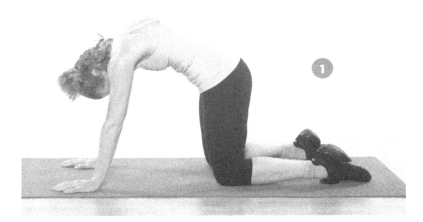

1 Inhale and draw your belly button in, causing your back to round.

2 Now exhale and slowly relax your body to the starting position.

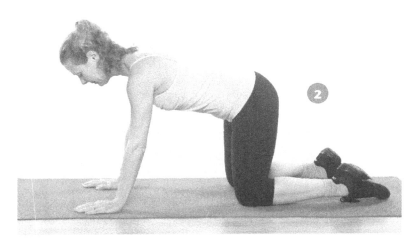

THE STRETCH: Sit on a mat with your knees bent and your feet flat on the floor. Place the soles of your feet together and gently allow your knees to drop to the floor. Place your hands on your ankles and gently pull yourself forward, not down. Hold this stretch for a comfortable moment.

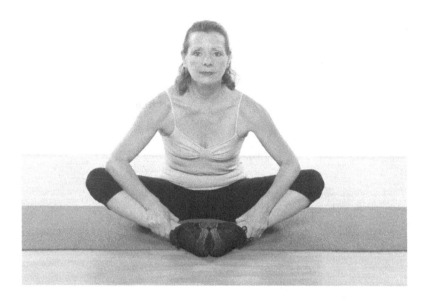

MODIFICATION: Loop a strap around your feet and gently pull yourself forward.

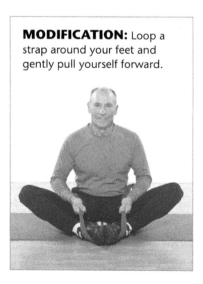

THE STRETCH: Sit on a mat with both legs extended into a V position and place both hands on the floor in front of you. Keep your head and torso tall, taking care not to round your back. Inhale and then exhale, allowing your weight to fall forward until you feel a comfortable stretch in the hamstrings and inner thighs. Hold this stretch for a comfortable moment, focusing on the sensation of the stretch, not on going as far as possible.

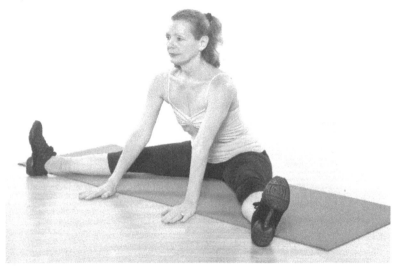

MODIFICATION: If you have trouble sitting up tall, try looping a strap around both feet.

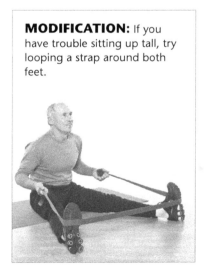

stretches
double knee to chest
target: low back, glutes

THE STRETCH: Lie on a mat and, if needed, place a pillow under your head. Bend your knees and hug them to your chest. Hold this position for a comfortable moment, feeling the stretch in your bottom and low back.

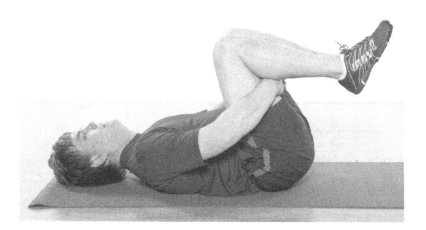

MODIFICATION: Loop a strap behind the backs of both legs and hold an end of the strap in each hand. Gently pull the straps to bring your knees to your chest.

VARIATION: This can also be done one leg at a time by extending one leg straight on the floor and using both hands to bring the other knee to your chest.

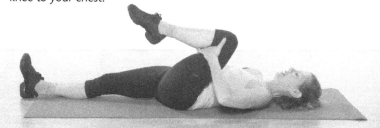

Caution: Avoid this stretch if you have hip problems.

THE STRETCH: Lie on a mat with both legs straight. Draw your left knee toward your right shoulder using your right hand. Hold for a comfortable moment, focusing on the sensation of the stretch, not on how close your knee comes to your shoulder.

Switch sides.

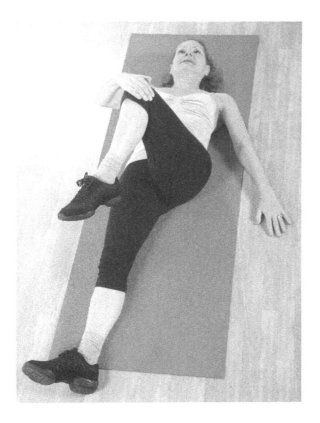

> **MODIFICATION:** You can also use a strap to help draw in your knee.

THE STRETCH: Lie on a mat with both legs straight. Using your left hand, gently bring your right knee across your center and toward your left side. Hold for a comfortable moment, focusing on the sensation of the stretch, not on how close your knee comes to the ground.

Switch sides.

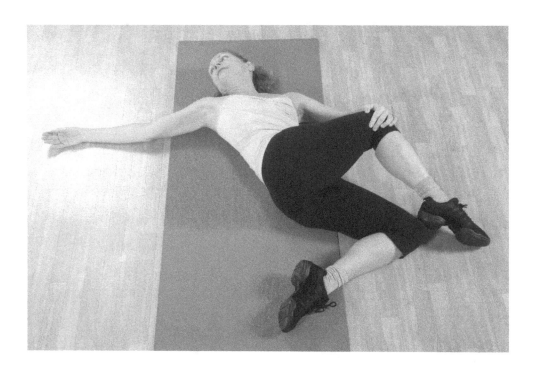

The piriformis muscle is a deep-lying muscle in the gluteal region, through which the sciatic nerve passes. When the piriformis is too tight, it can cramp the sciatic nerve, causing the symptoms of sciatica.

STARTING POSITION: Lie on a mat with your knees bent and your feet flat on the floor.

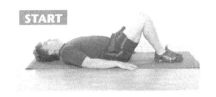

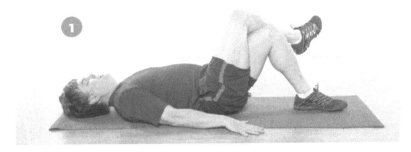

1 Cross your right knee on top of your left knee.

2 Place your hands under your left thigh and pull your knees in toward your chest. Stop when tension occurs. Hold this position for a comfortable moment, focusing on the sensation of the stretch.

Switch sides.

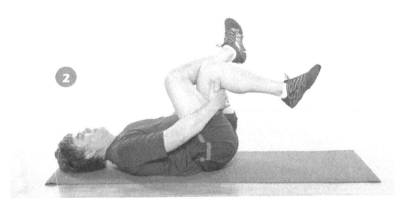

MODIFICATION: Loop a strap around both legs to assist in pulling in your knees.

STARTING POSITION: Stand with proper posture. Extend your right arm in front of you to shoulder height, with your palm facing forward and fingers pointing toward the ceiling.

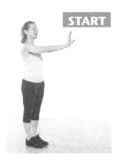

START

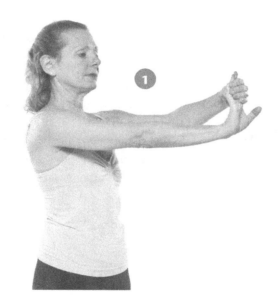

1 Gently pull your fingers back with your left hand until a desired stretch is felt under your wrist.

Hold the stretch for several seconds, then switch sides.

ADVANCED: Try doing the exercise with the fingertips pointing down.

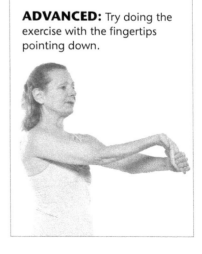

STARTING POSITION: Stand with proper posture.

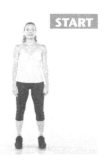

START

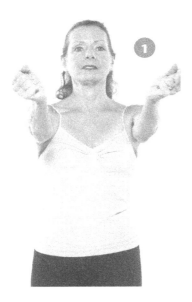

①

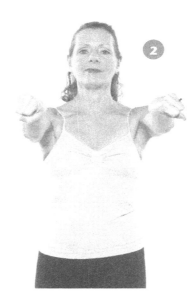

②

1–2 Raise both arms to shoulder height and slowly circle both wrists in both directions.

index

other books by karl knopf

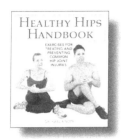

Healthy Hips Handbook
$14.95
Healthy Hips Handbook is designed to help prevent hip problems for some and, for those with existing hip problems, provide post-rehabilitation exercises.

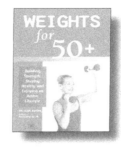

Weights for 50+
$14.95
Weight training is one of the most effective ways to get healthy and fight the physical signs of aging. *Weights for 50+* shows how easy it is for anyone to get started with weights.

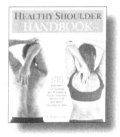

Healthy Shoulder Handbook
$14.95
Includes an overview of shoulder anatomy so anyone can use this friendly manual to strengthen an injured shoulder, identify the onset of a shoulder problem or better understand injury prevention.

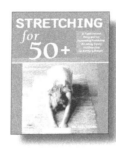

Stretching for 50+
$14.95
Based on the belief that individuals over 50 can do most of the same things as 20- and 30-year-olds, this book shows how to maintain and improve flexibility by incorporating stretching into one's life.

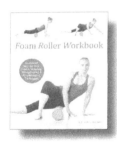

Foam Roller Workbook
$14.95
Details a comprehensive program for using the foam roller to recover from injury, reverse everyday pain and stay healthy in the future.

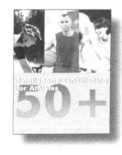

Total Sports Conditioning for Athletes 50+
$14.95
Provides sport-specific workouts that allow aging athletes to maintain the flexibility, strength and speed needed to win.

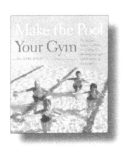

Make the Pool Your Gym
$14.95
Shows how to create an effective and efficient water workout that can build strength, improve cardiovascular fitness and burn calories.

To order these books call 800-377-2542 or 510-601-8301, fax 510-601-8307, e-mail ulysses@ulyssespress.com, or write to Ulysses Press, P.O. Box 3440, Berkeley, CA 94703. All retail orders are shipped free of charge. California residents must include sales tax. Allow two to three weeks for delivery.

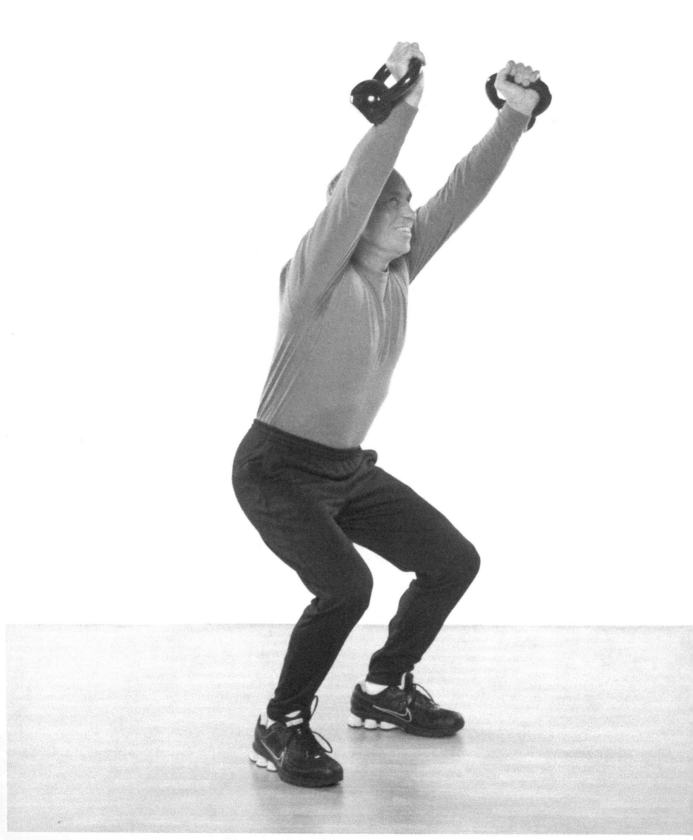

acknowledgments

A special thanks goes to Lily Chou for sharing her insights and knowledge about kettlebells, which significantly improved the outcome of this book. Additionally, a giant thank you to the models, Toni Silver and Rob Harrison, as well as Fred Brevold, who served as both a model and an advisor. Much appreciation also to the skilled photographic team at Rapt Productions. Lastly, a special thanks goes to my son Chris Knopf, who allowed me to experiment some modification techniques on him.

about the author

KARL KNOPF, author of *Foam Roller Workbook*, *Healthy Hips Handbook*, *Healthy Shoulder Handbook*, *Make the Pool Your Gym*, *Stretching for 50+*, *Weights for 50+* and *Total Sports Conditioning for Athletes 50+*, has been involved with the health and fitness of the disabled and older adults for 35 years. A consultant on numerous National Institutes of Health grants, Knopf has served as advisor to the PBS exercise series *Sit and Be Fit* and to the State of California on disabilities issues. He is a frequent speaker at conferences and has written several textbooks and articles. Knopf coordinates the Fitness Therapist Program at Foothill College in Los Altos Hills, California.

CPSIA information can be obtained
at www.ICGtesting.com
Printed in the USA
JSHW011123110820
7221JS00004B/22